The Diabetic's Healthy Exchanges® Cookbook

G·K Hall &Co.

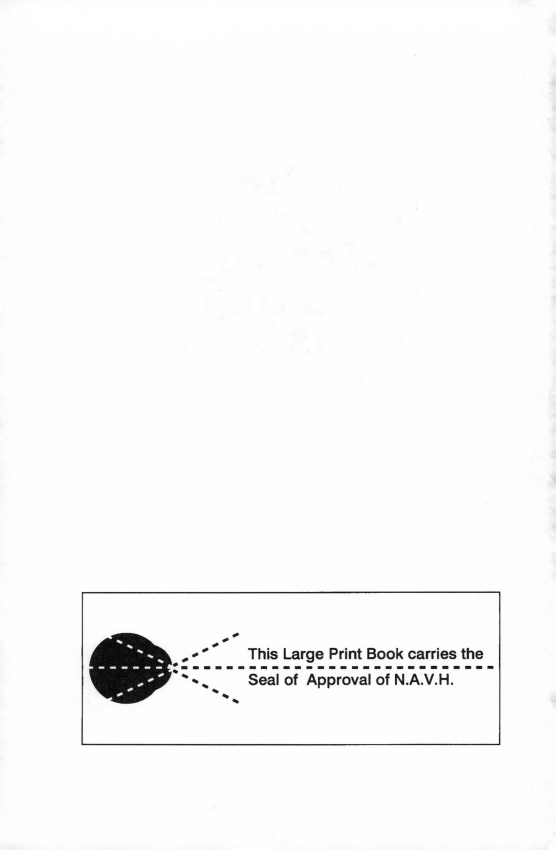

This Large Print Book carries the
Seal of Approval of N.A.V.H.

The Diabetic's Healthy Exchanges® Cookbook

JoAnna M. Lund

Introduction by
Janet Meirelles, R.N., B.S.N., C.D.E.

Diabetic Exchanges Calculated by
Rose Hoenig, R.D., L.D.

G.K. Hall & Co.
Thorndike, Maine

Published in 1997 by arrangement with Perigee Books, an imprint of The Berkley Publishing Group.

G.K. Hall Large Print Reference Collection.

The text of this Large Print edition is unabridged. Other aspects of the book may vary from the original edition.

Set in 16 pt. Plantin by Juanita Macdonald.

Printed in the United States on permanent paper.

Library of Congress Cataloging in Publication Data

Lund, JoAnna M.
    The diabetic's healthy exchanges cookbook / JoAnna M. Lund ; introduction by Janet Meirelles ; diabetic exchanges calculated by Rose Hoenig. — [Thorndike large print ed.]
      p.   cm.
    Originally published by New York : Perigee Books, 1996.
    Includes index.
    ISBN 0-7838-8199-1 (lg. print : hc : alk. paper)
    1. Diabetes — Diet therapy — Recipes.   I. Title.
[RC662.L86   1997]
641.5´6314—dc21   97-11521

As all my books are, this cookbook is dedicated in loving memory to my parents, Jerome and Agnes McAndrews. It is also dedicated to all those who must watch their diets because of diabetes. Both my parents developed adult-onset diabetes, and I saw the pleasure go out of their meals as they had to learn to cook and eat differently. Oh, how I wish I could have shared my delicious recipes in this book with them. They would have enjoyed them so much.

I hope that by my sharing these "common folk" healthy recipes with you, many of the dishes will become traditions in your home and that you'll proudly share them with family and friends. When you do, please thank my parents, as the creative ability to develop the recipes and the analytical skills required to make the exchanges come out right are talents I inherited from them.

When you question why you have to cook and eat differently because of medical concerns, please read the poem on the following page my mother composed. The reason she wrote it was a broken ankle, but the message is appropriate for any new circumstance we must face in our lives.

Why

Why this new cross was given to me,
    I wasn't sure.
Wearing a heavy cast was more than
    I thought I could endure.
At first, it was hard to accept and I
    was so sad and blue.
Then the reason was revealed,
    and I suddenly knew.
It really was a blessing in disguise in
    so many ways.
And I will be thankful to God for
    the rest of my days.
Never again will I question what is
    expected of me to bear.
Instead, I will ask Him for help,
    then leave the rest in His care.

— Agnes Carrington McAndrews

Contents

Acknowledgments

When I set out to solve a problem for me and my family, I never dreamed that I would also be solving problems for so many other families as well. I can't begin to count the times that people with diabetes have told me how I have brought pleasure back into their lives because my food tastes so good. But no matter how good my recipes are, I never could have spread the message to so many without the support and help of some very special people. For helping me to help myself and in the process help others, I want to express my thanks:

To all the doctors and registered dietitians who saw the validity of my recipes and recommended them to their patients.

To Rose Hoenig, R.D., L.D., for computing the diabetic exchanges and answering my questions about healthy nutrition.

To Janet Meirelles, R.N., B.S.N., C.D.E., for helping to explain the nutritional needs for those with diabetes.

To Becky, James, Tommy, Pam, John, Zach, Josh, Mary, Regina, Marge, Cleland, and Catherine — my family. From my two-year-old grandchild to my ninety-year-old aunt, they all gladly taste test my Healthy Exchanges creations.

To Angela Miller and Coleen O'Shea, my agents. They enjoy helping me "stir up" new ideas for cookbooks.

To Barbara Alpert, my writing associate. She willingly visits with me via the phone when I need to share ideas with her — even at 5:00 A.M.

To John Duff, my editor. He encourages me to continue creating recipes and never tries to change me or my "common folk" healthy way of cooking.

To Phyllis Grann, Susan Petersen, Barbara O'Shea, Judy Miller, Fern Edison, Donna Gould, and everyone at Perigee Books for supporting me as I continue to write cookbooks. Who would have ever believed that this middle-aged grandmother could be an author for such a prestigious publisher!

To Cliff Lund, my husband and "official taste-tester." He's always loved me no matter what size my hips were. As Healthy Exchanges continues to take on a life of its own, he still gives me his unconditional support and love. He truly is, as the popular song lyrics say, "the wind beneath my wings."

To God, for giving me the talent to create "common folk" healthy recipes and the courage to share my past so that I may help others with their future.

Introduction

Your physician just told you that you have diabetes. Does this mean you can never eat pie again?

Your husband's doctor told him his Type II diabetes would improve if he would lose some weight and cut down on sweets. Does this mean no more lasagna or gooey dessert?

Your six-year-old granddaughter has Type I diabetes. Does this mean you have to hide the cookies when she visits?

Your friend and co-worker has developed diabetes during her pregnancy. Does that mean you can never bring another cake to an office party?

The answer to all these questions is No!

You and your loved ones don't have to give up dessert, you don't have to buy your food in the dietetic section of your supermarket, and you don't have to watch every morsel that goes in your or their mouths.

Understanding the types of diabetes and how you can effectively manage each type — especially through diet — will help you to reduce many of the complications of diabetes. But you do not have to give up all your favorite foods. With the help of people like JoAnna Lund, anyone can enjoy a full and active life without the kind of sacrifices that once made managing diabetes so difficult.

Different Types of Diabetes and Their Causes

Type I:

Type I diabetes, also known as juvenile-onset diabetes or Insulin Dependent Diabetes Mellitus (IDDM), occurs in less than ten percent of people with diabetes. Type I diabetics *must* take at least two insulin injections a day. They also benefit from a closely regulated diet, especially monitoring the amounts of carbohydrates, eating at regular times and taking extra precautions when exercising.

Type II:

Type II diabetes is also commonly called adult-onset diabetes or Non-insulin Dependent Diabetes Mellitus (NIDDM). Ninety percent of the people with diabetes have Type II and at least eighty percent of these people are overweight and relatively inactive. It seems that the excess body fat many of us pad ourselves with after we turn forty or so causes a resistance to our own insulin production that may result in diabetes.

In many cases, people with Type II can keep their blood sugar in the normal range (80–120 mg/dl) by regular exercise and some modification in their eating, such as reducing the amount of sugar and other carbohydrates (like bread, noodles, rice, etc.) in their diet and eating smaller meals more frequently throughout the day. About one-third of those with Type II must also take oral medication (these oral medications are not pill forms of insulin) to lower blood sugar; the other one-third need insulin shots.

Gestational:

Gestational diabetes occurs when the pregnancy hormones in the body make insulin less effective. Uncontrolled blood sugar may contribute to a premature or difficult birth or a very big baby (over nine pounds), which may also suffer from long-lasting effects including heart defects and respiratory problems. By maintaining a proper diet, especially by reducing the amount of foods that contain carbohydrates, or in some cases taking insulin injections (oral diabetes medications are not good for the baby), the gestational diabetic patient can keep blood sugar in the normal range and minimize or eliminate any adverse effect.

Fortunately, gestational diabetes almost always goes away as soon as the baby is born. However, women who have had this condition have a fifty percent greater risk of getting Type II diabetes within ten years. They can improve their chances of not eventually becoming permanently diabetic by maintaining their weight in the normal range with sensible eating and regular exercise.

What Diabetics Have in Common

Although different types of diabetes require different management, the common problem in all types is that the amount of sugar (glucose) in the blood exceeds normal levels.

In Type I diabetes, the insulin-producing cells in the pancreas (a gland near the stomach) have been destroyed. Scientists believe the cells are probably killed by an over-reaction of the immune system to a virus in susceptible people.

Without insulin to "unlock" cells, glucose from food accumulates in the blood. The result is thicker, stickier blood that damages nerves and blood vessels, causing the complications that occur in people with diabetes. Also, if the glucose stays in the blood vessels, the cells that need it are deprived of their food, so they can't function and may eventually start dying.

In Type II diabetes, the pancreas continues to produce insulin, but for some reason this insulin doesn't "unlock" enough of the cells to adequately feed them and to keep the blood sugar in the normal range.

Gestational diabetes is very similar to Type II diabetes — the pancreas produces insulin, but pregnancy hormones prevent it from working effectively.

The goal of any treatment for diabetes is to maintain blood-sugar levels in the normal range. Higher than normal blood-sugar levels may result in nerve and blood vessel damage. Not enough glucose in the blood results in shakiness, sweatiness, confusion, and, if not corrected promptly, coma, or even death.

Food, or more correctly, the *right* food at the

right time in the *right* amounts is the first step in managing diabetes. Without sensible eating, almost nothing else in the doctor's "bag" will make much difference.

What people with diabetes ought to eat, and ought not to eat, is often misunderstood. Even if you know what is sensible and what isn't, you'll meet people who *don't* know but *think they do*. Some of the most common myths about food and diabetes are:

Myth #1: Sugar *must* always be avoided.

Myth #2: Artificial sweeteners are dangerous.

Myth #3: Fat is OK.

Myth #4: Fiber is only important for treating constipation.

Myth #5: Snacks are optional.

Myth #6: Eating on time is good, but not essential.

Myth #1: Sugar Must Always Be Avoided.

Since the body changes many of the foods we eat into sugar, the total elimination of sugar from the diet is impossible. Candy and desserts aren't the only things that raise our blood sugar. All of the carbohydrates we eat, about half of the protein, and even about ten percent of the fat in our food is transformed into glucose in our digestive tract.

Carbohydrate (sugar and starch) foods include

ones you may not even have considered starchy. Corn, peas, beans, and other legumes are more like bread than vegetables. And milk contains more sugar than protein, so it's also considered a breadlike food to people with diabetes.

Here, for example, is the nutritional content label from a container of nonfat, artificially sweetened yogurt:

Nutrition Facts

Serving Size 1 Container (227 g)

Amount per Serving
Calories 100 Calories from Fat 0
Total Fat 0 g
Saturated Fat 0 g
Cholesterol less than 5 mg
Sodium 140 mg
Potassium 480 mg
Total Carbohydrate 17 g
Dietary Fiber 0 g
Sugars 15 g*
Protein 9 g

* Sugar was not added to the yogurt. This is the sugar — lactose — naturally found in milk.

Diabetic Exchanges

The sample label above gives nutritional information in grams — a lot of grams. But instead of giving you nutritional goals in hundreds of grams of carbohydrate, for example, dietitians usually recommend the number of *diabetic exchanges* you should eat at each meal. "Exchanges" are rather like "dozens" or "tons" or other collective words; they allow you to think in more manageable numbers.

In the diabetic exchange system for meal planning, foods are grouped together in "exchange groups." Each serving of a food in each category has a certain number of grams of carbohydrate, protein and/or fat and a certain number of calories.

The groups are called exchanges because, *in the specified amounts,* each food within an exchange group can be exchanged for another in the same group. A more extensive discussion of diabetic exchanges begins on page 40.

New Recommendations for Diabetics

Until recently, nutritionists believed that granulated sugar, honey, corn syrup, molasses, and foods containing them had to be limited more carefully than complex carbohydrates, such as bread, potatoes, pasta, rice, and beans. However, several recent research studies have shown that when eaten with a meal, *sugar does not raise blood sugar more than a starchy food with an equal amount of carbohydrate.*

Because we now know that *the total grams of carbohydrate in a meal* are more important than whether some of those carbohydrates are simple sugars, in 1995 the American Diabetes Association combined the old bread/starch, fruit, vegetable, and milk exchange groups into one group, labeled the "Carbohydrate Group."

Nowadays, a dietitian is unlikely to recommend a breakfast with two bread exchanges, one fruit exchange, and one milk exchange. With the *revised exchange* lists, you would be instructed to choose, for example, any four breads, OR four fruits, OR four milks, OR any combination of the three as long as the total amount of carbohydrate added up to about 60 grams. *And,* some of that 60 grams could be granulated sugar, or honey, or any of the formerly "forbidden" sweeteners. However, sugar, honey, etc., are *concentrated sweeteners. Very small amounts add up to a lot of carbohydrates in a hurry.* For instance, 3 teaspoons of granulated sugar have the same amount of carbohydrate as 3 cups of popcorn.

You probably would agree with me that 3 cups of popcorn is more satisfying than that little bit of sugar — which is why, despite the new evidence about sugar, most people with diabetes still limit their sugar intake. It is possible, though, for them to have a piece of birthday cake or other sweet treat without raising their blood sugar — IF they trade their potatoes, bread, and/or starchy vegetable (corn, peas, etc.) for the carbohydrates in the cake.

Clearly, it would not be a good idea to do this very often: potatoes, bread, and starchy vegetables have fiber, protein, and vitamins and minerals that sugar doesn't have. But it *is* possible that what you see on your diabetic friend's plate that looks to you like forbidden food, was actually traded for other carbohydrates.

The good news is that new technology has managed to make many more foods very low in fat and low in sugar.

Myth #2: Artificial Sweeteners Are Dangerous.

There is no scientific evidence that even long-term use of artificial sweeteners causes any health problems (unless you are specifically allergic). Repeated double-blind studies (where neither the researcher nor the subject knew what was in a capsule, aspartame or a placebo) have not shown that aspartame causes any change in body chemistry. Several long-term studies published in such respected medical journals as the *New England Journal of Medicine*, the *Archives of Internal Medicine*, and *The Journal of Allergy and Clinical Immunology* have demonstrated that aspartame has no effect on hunger, while one showed greater weight loss in a dieting group that used aspartame.

Aspartame is made from two protein building blocks that are present in large quantities naturally in foods such as bananas. The evidence that aspartame is safe to use is so convincing that dietitians routinely recommend it even for women who have gestational diabetes.

Cyclamate failed the FDA's safety requirements in tests on lab animals and was banned in 1970 in the U.S. However, in every other country in the world cyclamate continued to be used without any reported problems.

Saccharin (the chemical in Sweet 'n Low, Sugar Twin, and other artificial sweeteners) also failed to meet FDA safety standards in the '70s, but because it was the only sugar-free, calorie-free artificial sweetener left on the market, American dieters and diabetics pressured the FDA to permit its continued sale. It's still used in the U.S. and the rest of the world without reports of negative health effects, except on laboratory rats who got bladder cancer when given huge doses of saccharin.

Acesulfame K (found in Sweet One) has not been on the market as long as saccharin, cyclamate, or aspartame, but it has been approved by the FDA and has been available for several years in the U.S.

Artificial Sweeteners Compared

Sweetener	Stays Sweet When Heated	Aftertaste
Aspartame (Equal)	no	no
Saccharin (Sugar Twin)	yes	may be bitter
Acesulfame K (Sweet One)	yes	no
Cyclamate (not available in the U.S.)	yes	no

Sugar does more than just sweeten our food. It adds body to ingredients and holds in moisture. None of the artificial sweeteners can do this, so you usually can't replace all the sugar in a recipe with the equivalent amount of artificial sweetener, especially not in baked goods. (The makers of Sweet One state that you can substitute up to one-half of the sugar called for in a recipe with Sweet One without the texture suffering too much.)

In this book some of the recipes have been devised to use Equal (which would normally lose its sweetness when heated), even in a dish that requires cooking. In these recipes the food is cooked first and Equal is added only after the cooking is complete.

Even though artificial sweeteners aren't perfect, you can use them to replace some of the sugar in recipes. Also, when you use artificial sweeteners, you can have larger portions than you could with sugar-sweetened foods.

Myth #3: Fat Is O.K.

Before the discovery of insulin in 1922, people with diabetes could literally "starve to death" because they could not process carbohydrates. Therefore, the recommended diet, albeit unsuccessful in the long run, was one that eliminated carbohydrates and emphasized high fat as a source of calories.

The medical management of diabetes today may include insulin therapy, but it inevitably calls for reducing fat in the diet in order to reduce the incidence of cardiovascular disease, which can lead to heart attack and stroke. Strokes and heart attacks are two to seven times more common in people with diabetes than in the general population because too much sugar in the blood damages vessels and nerves. Also, cholesterol and triglycerides (another type of fat found in the blood) are frequently too high with diabetes, and clog arteries even more. Since cardiovascular disease is partly hereditary, you can't control *all* the factors that cause it, but you *can* control many factors that increase your chances of getting it.

The first line of defense is avoiding the foods that clog arteries, including those with cholesterol, triglycerides, and saturated fat.

Is Butter Really So Bad?
Is Margarine Better?

Although you may have given up butter in favor of margarine to eliminate cholesterol, margarine's negative characteristic is the presence of trans-fatty acids.

In order to change liquid vegetable oil (which has no cholesterol) into semisolid margarine, food processors saturate the oil with hydrogen. The result is a partially hydrogenated oil with trans-fatty acids.

Evidence shows that trans-fatty acids may promote heart disease. Some researchers also suspect that trans-fatty acids may retard fetal growth (one study showed that expectant mothers who ate higher levels of trans-fatty acids had smaller babies with smaller head circumferences). While there is no definitive proof for either of these consequences of eating margarine or shortening with trans-fatty acids, a prudent strategy is to eat only small amounts of margarine, shortening, or butter. In short, eat less saturated fat, period.

The recipes in this book call for very small amounts of fat, especially saturated fat (which your body uses as a raw material to make cholesterol). When possible, use canola oil or olive oil for cooking and cut down on foods that are high in saturated fat and/or trans-fatty acids.

How Will You Know What Has Saturated Fat and Trans-Fatty Acids?

Look on food labels for buzzwords such as *"partially hydrogenated [any kind of] oil"* and ask fast-food restaurants for nutritional information — many of them have printed materials you can read at your leisure.

In short, if you reduce your intake of foods that contain fat to small amounts, you'll be cutting saturated fat along with cholesterol, AND you'll slash calories.

Myth #4: Fiber Is Only Important for Treating Constipation.

Fiber is much, much more than an aid to staying regular.

Fiber's benefits include:

- increasing the effectiveness of insulin

- delaying and smoothing the absorption of sugars from the digestive tract

- lowering cholesterol and triglyceride levels

- lowering blood pressure

- promoting weight loss (by making you feel full longer after eating)

- helping prevent colon, breast, and ovarian cancers

- helping prevent diverticulosis and hemorrhoids

Fiber is available *only from plant foods*. (There's no fiber in meat, for example, no matter how chewy it is). To get enough fiber, eat at least eleven to twenty servings of vegetables, fruits, beans, and grain foods every day. (The number of servings depends on how much food you eat. Big, active men would need twenty.) Six to ten of those servings should be from fruits and vegetables — you're aiming for 25–35 grams of fiber daily (some sources even recommend 40–50 grams a day).

Do six to ten servings of fruits and vegetables and five to ten servings of bread, rice, pasta, and potatoes seem unattainable? It's easier than you think, because what's considered a serving is quite a small portion. For example, an average-size orange is equal to two fruit servings; most bananas are two fruit servings; a serving of cooked vegetables that is only ½ cup equals one serving; one bagel equals two to four bread servings, and ⅓ cup of rice equals one bread serving.

An adequate daily intake of fiber could be reached if you ate the following:

Exchanges/Servings	Food
1½ bread	1 cup cooked oatmeal
2 fruit	1 medium orange
2 bread	2 slices bread (sandwich)
1 bread, 2 vegetable	1 cup bean soup
2 vegetable	¾ cup carrot salad
2 bread	1 cup cooked spaghetti
2 vegetable	½ cup marinara sauce
1 fruit	½ cup canned pears (in juice, not syrup)

Here are the totals:
 9 fruit and vegetable servings
 6½ bread servings
 860 calories

Even if you were trying to limit your total daily calories to 1,500, there's still room left for lean meat, beverages, etc.

Get your fiber from more than one source to be sure you're getting sufficient soluble AND insoluble fiber. Both have benefits.

Soluble fiber is found in significant quantities in oat bran, oatmeal, beans, and psyllium (found in fiber supplements such as Metamucil). It reduces triglycerides and cholesterol — and much more.

Insoluble fiber is found in whole grains and

vegetables. It's especially good for the gastrointestinal system.

One of the best ways to get a head start on providing yourself and your loved ones with enough fiber is to start your day with a high-fiber cereal. You might be able to get half your fiber from your breakfast cereal — but not if you think the name of the cereal or the claims on the *front* of cereal boxes are always accurate. If you do, you'll get lots of crunch but probably not much fiber. What you really need to know is found in the nutritional information on the side of the box. Check the nutrition label for "dietary fiber" content (it's in the carbohydrate category). **Cereals with a total of at least 8 grams per serving are significant sources of fiber.**

Some cereals give you little fiber for your calories. An example is granola-type cereals. These can contain as much fat as a pat of butter *in a mere ounce.*

Here are some other sources of fiber (especially soluble fiber):

Fiber per 100 Calories

	Total Grams	% of Total That's Soluble	Grams of Soluble Fiber
black-eyed peas	4.4	46	2.0
kidney beans	5.5	29	1.6
red beans	7.0	29	2.0
prunes	3.0	29	0.9
corn	2.5	45	1.1
carrots	7.4	48	3.6
peas	4.9	51	2.5

Myth #5: Snacks Are Optional.

Snacks are essential to someone with diabetes who takes a medicine that lowers blood sugar. It's not unusual for a dietitian to recommend **3 meals and 3 snacks a day**. These snacks keep blood sugar from dipping too low between meals or when exercise has used up the available glucose.

People with diabetes are encouraged to carry some form of sugar *at all times*. In addition, they often have crackers and other foods to hold them over if they're caught in traffic or can't eat on schedule for some other reason.

An especially important snack is at bedtime. The bedtime snack helps keep blood sugar at normal levels throughout the night. Many people with

Type II diabetes who are overweight are tempted to skip their bedtime snack to save calories.

For those who want to lose weight, skipping a snack is not the solution. Under the guidance of a nutrition consultant, you can reduce portion sizes throughout the day and make other changes that will maintain blood sugar at normal levels, despite fewer total calories and carbohydrates overall.

Myth #6: Eating on Time Is Good, but Not Essential.

Timing of meals and snacks is important to anyone who takes insulin or oral medications to lower blood sugar. Many diabetes medications are designed to act over long periods of time with a significant blood sugar lowering effect *hours after* they are taken. The medicines keep working even when the last meal's food has been absorbed. If there's no new food to restock the blood with sugar, cells will go without food. This is most critical to the brain and explains why so many of the symptoms of moderately low blood sugar are related to brain cell malfunction: confusion, lack of coordination, slurred speech, seizures, and losing consciousness.

It's important for diabetics to be able to predict when the medication will peak and to eat at about that time. One of the most common complaints I hear from patients and my friends with diabetes is "Other people don't take me seriously when I say I need to eat between five and six. They tell me to 'chill out,' or 'take it easy, dinner'll be ready in a while.' "

When food is late, the diabetic must snack. This seems to offer a simple solution to delayed meals, but remember that the carbohydrates and calories eaten for the snack will need to be subtracted from the meal.

Cooking for Someone with Diabetes
If you have diabetes or regularly cook for someone with diabetes, you will find the advice of a dietitian very helpful. You'll learn how to choose foods you like in the right portions to reach your (or your loved one's) weight, blood sugar and cholesterol goals. A qualified dietitian will help with timing of meals, snacks, exercise, and medication.

Cooking for Guests with Diabetes
One of my diabetic friends was embarrassed at a dinner party when the hostess announced to everyone at the dining table that she prepared my friend's food by following a diabetes cookbook. The hostess's heart was in the right place but my friend would have preferred to have had what everybody else was served. If something was not on her meal plan, she could have had a tiny taste and left the rest.

At my last buffet party, I had little notes stuck to serving platters that said things like "fat-free bean dip" and "sugar-free" by the whipped topping and pumpkin pie. It didn't look very elegant but it did the job.

It used to be that serving healthier foods took more time and trouble. It is more time consuming to choose, wash, cut up, and display a tray of veggies than to dump out a bag of chips and open a container of fatty sour cream dip.

Fortunately, you can now buy ready-to-eat vegetables, salad greens, and fruit salad at many supermarkets and, of course, there is a wide array of sugar-free, low-fat products readily available.

You don't have to make separate meals for your guests with diabetes. Actually, the dishes you can make with JoAnna Lund's recipes will delight *every* guest, and no one will even know they're meant to be healthy.

What to Serve to Drink

Sugar-free sodas will be appreciated by most diabetics. Beware when shopping, however. There are some flavored sparkling waters and clear sodas that are sweetened with high-fructose corn syrup. Many have almost as much sugar and calories as regular soda pop. *Check the label carefully* for ingredients and look for a drink that is *artificially* sweetened.

For the occasional diabetic who does not want an artificially sweetened beverage, serving tomato juice or V-8 makes a good alternative provided the sodium content is not too high.

What About Alcohol?

If you have diabetes and you take insulin or other medicine to lower your blood sugar, drinking alcohol can be risky. Alcohol can lead to severely low blood sugars if taken without a meal or "to excess" even with food. That's because the liver, which gives us emergency sugar when we haven't eaten for a while, gets too busy processing the alcohol to release stored sugar. Without sugar from food OR the liver, blood sugar can get very low. And even if you only drink alcoholic beverages with dinner, you could still get low blood sugar hours after you've digested your meal. If that low blood sugar occurs when you're sleeping (or driving), you could become unconscious before you could take steps (eat or drink sugary food) to help yourself.

There's more bad news — new research shows that more than 4 ounces of alcohol *a week* (that's not a misprint, I really mean 4 ounces alcohol within 7 days) accelerates nerve damage. That damage is called neuropathy and is responsible for most of the foot and leg amputations, all too common in folks with diabetes.

In addition to the health issue, alcohol has a surprisingly high number of calories, almost as many as fat. One and a half ounces of hard liquor, 4 ounces of wine, or 12 ounces of beer each have the equivalent of two fat exchanges or 90 calories from the alcohol portion alone. Wine and beer have still more calories from the carbohydrate they also contain.

Drinking alcohol can also impair your judgment and make you forget your diet and pile on the wrong foods.

Taking Care of Diabetes Brings Healthy Changes

You may have to change some long-entrenched habits, in exchange for a longer, healthier and more energetic life.

To control your blood glucose and lower your risk of heart disease, these are sensible goals:

- cut down on sugar and other concentrated carbohydrates (honey, corn syrup, etc.)
- lose weight or continue to maintain a sensible weight
- cut down on fat, especially saturated fat
- eat more vegetables, fruits, and whole grains
- substitute non-fat dairy products for high-fat ones
- eat smaller meals, at more regular times
- get at least 25, preferably 40, grams of fiber every day
- eat all snacks recommended for you by your dietitian
- exercise at least 30 minutes a day, every day
- stay informed about new health-improving discoveries.

My patients and friends with diabetes tell me it's worth the effort. They say that keeping their blood sugar under control makes them feel ten years younger.

Since you'll be thinking about what to eat at least three times a day, it's nice to have a cookbook (like this one) of delicious, healthy, and quick-to-make dishes — it's so much easier to make sensible choices when you don't have to give up your favorite foods.

Take care of yourself and your diabetes — and *bon appetit!*

— Janet Meirelles, R.N., B.S.N., C.H.E.S., C.D.E.
Author, *Diabetes Is Not a Piece of Cake*

How I Learned to Help Myself

JoAnna M. Lund and Healthy Exchanges

For twenty-eight years I was the diet queen of DeWitt, Iowa. I tried every diet I ever heard of, every one I could afford, and every one that found its way to my small town in eastern Iowa. I was willing to try anything that promised to "melt off the pounds," determined to deprive my body in every possible way in order to become thin at last.

I sent away for expensive "miracle" diet pills. I starved myself on the Cambridge Diet and the Bahama Diet. I gobbled Ayds diet candies, took thyroid pills, fiber pills, prescription and over-the-counter diet pills. I went to endless weight-loss support-group meetings, but I managed to take healthy programs such as Overeaters Anonymous, Weight Watchers, and TOPS and turn them into unhealthy diets . . . diets I could never follow for more than a few months.

I was determined to discover something that worked long-term, but each new failure increased my desperation that I'd never find it.

I ate strange concoctions and rubbed on even stranger potions. I tried liquid diets like Slim•Fast ™ and Metrecal. I agreed to be hypnotized. I tried reflexology and even had an acupuncture device stuck in my ear!

Does my story sound a lot like yours? I'm not surprised. No wonder the weight-loss business is a billion-dollar industry!

Every new thing I tried seemed to work — at least at first. And losing that first five or ten pounds would get me so excited, I'd believe that this new miracle diet would finally get my weight off for keeps.

Inevitably, though, the initial excitement wore off. The diet's routine and boredom set in, and I quit. I shoved the pills to the back of the medicine chest, pushed the cans of powdered shake mix to the rear of the kitchen cabinets, slid all the program materials out of sight under my bed, and once more felt like a failure.

Like most dieters, I quickly gained back the weight I'd lost each time, along with a few extra "souvenir" pounds that seemed always to settle around my hips. I'd done the diet-lose-weight-gain-it-all-back "yo-yo" on the average of once a year. It's no exaggeration to say that over the years I've lost 1,000 pounds — and gained back 1,150 pounds.

Finally, at the age of forty-six I weighed more than I'd ever imagined possible. I'd stopped believing that any diet could work for me. I drowned my sorrows in sacks of cake donuts and wondered if I'd live long enough to watch my grandchildren grow up.

Something had to change.

I had to change.

Finally, I did.

I'm just over fifty now — and I'm 130 pounds less than my all-time high of close to 300 pounds. I've kept the weight off for more than five years. I'd like to lose another ten pounds, but I'm not obsessed about it. If it takes me two or three years to accomplish it, that's okay.

What I *do* care about is never saying hello again to any of those unwanted pounds I said good-bye to!

How did I jump off the roller coaster I was on? For one thing, I finally stopped looking to food to solve my emotional problems. But what really shook me up — and got me started on the path that changed my life — was Operation Desert Storm in early 1991. I sent three children off to the Persian Gulf war — my son-in-law, Matt, a medic in Special Forces; my daughter, Becky, a full-time college student and member of a medical unit in the Army Reserve; and my son James, a member of the Inactive Army Reserve but reactivated as a chemicals expert.

Somehow, knowing that my children were putting their lives on the line got me thinking about my own mortality — and I knew in my heart the last thing they needed while they were overseas was to get a letter from home saying that their mother was ill because of a food-related problem.

The day I drove the third child to the airport to leave for Saudi Arabia, something happened to me that would change my life for the better —

and forever. I stopped praying my constant prayer as a professional dieter, which was simply "Please, God, let me lose ten pounds by Friday." Instead, I began praying, "God, please help me not to be a burden to my kids and my family."

I quit praying for what I wanted, and started praying for what I needed — and, in the process, my prayers were answered. I couldn't keep the kids safe — that was out of my hands — but I could try to get healthier to better handle the stress of it. It was the least I could do on the home front.

That quiet prayer was the beginning of the new JoAnna Lund. My initial goal was not to lose weight or create healthy recipes. I only wanted to become healthier for my kids, my husband, and myself.

Each of my children returned safely from the Persian Gulf. But something didn't come back — the 130 extra pounds I'd been lugging around for far too long. I'd finally accepted the truth after all those agonizing years of suffering through on-again, off-again dieting.

There are no "magic" cures in life.

No "magic" potion, pill, or diet will make unwanted pounds disappear.

I found something better than magic, if you can believe it. When I turned my weight and health dilemma over to God for guidance, a new JoAnna Lund and Healthy Exchanges were born.

I discovered a new way to live my life — and uncovered an unexpected talent for creating easy "common folk" healthy recipes, and sharing my commonsense approach to healthy living. I learned that I could motivate others to change their lives and adopt a positive outlook. I began publishing cookbooks and a monthly food newsletter, and speaking to groups all over the country.

I like to say, *"When life handed me a lemon, not only did I make healthy, tasty lemonade, I wrote the recipe down!"*

What I finally found was not a quick fix or a short-term diet but a great way to live well for a lifetime.

I want to share it with you.

What Healthy Exchanges Means

Is it really possible to enjoy favorite foods once the excess sugars and fats are removed? Yes, and I can prove it to you — just as I proved to myself and my family that I could create healthy recipes that tasted like "real food."

When I came up with the concept for Healthy Exchanges, I had three ideas in mind:

1. I wanted to **"exchange"** old, unhealthy habits for new, healthy ones in food, exercise, and mental attitude.

2. I chose to **"exchange"** ingredients within each recipe to eliminate as much fat and sugar as possible, while retaining the original flavor, appearance, and aroma.

3. I calculated all recipes using the **exchange** system of measuring daily food intake as established by the American Dietetic Association, the American Diabetic Association, and many national weight-loss organizations.

The Diabetic's Healthy Exchanges Cookbook can help you accomplish your healthy living goals, whatever they are. Maybe you need to stabilize your blood sugar. Maybe you need to lower your cholesterol. Maybe you want to eat healthily. Or maybe you need to lose a few pounds — or a few more than that. But you need to find delicious, easy-to-make recipes the rest of the family will eat without objection. The dieter or health-conscious person may be willing to accept uninspired, low-fat, low-sugar "diet" recipes — but what can you do when your kids want pizza and your husband insists on hot fudge sundaes and pie?

Most diet recipes deserve their bad reputations. Too many of them sacrifice taste and appeal for lower calories and less sodium or sweetener. That's usually why nobody likes to eat them — and why even if we stick to this kind of eating for a while, we eventually jump off the wagon!

This book will change that — and change it for good. Ever since I began creating recipes, I aimed for what I call "common-folk healthy" — meaning that the recipes I create have to fit into an already busy lifestyle, they have to consider our likes and dislikes as a family, and they have to appeal to everyone sitting at my table.

I do not shop at health-food stores, and I don't like preparing complicated dishes that keep me in the kitchen for hours. I got tired of being left with a pile of dirty dishes to show for all my efforts once the family had bolted from the table after a mere ten minutes. People may laugh when I say, If it takes longer to fix it than it does to eat it, forget it — but you'll be amazed to discover that you can eat well *and* healthily without spending hours cooking, chopping, and cleaning up!

My goal is this: The foods that I prepare have

to look, taste, smell, and feel like the foods we have always enjoyed. Because I figured out how to "exchange" the excess fats and sugars within each recipe with readily available healthy ingredients, you'll be able to enjoy "real-food" dishes like pizza, mashed potatoes, and cherry cheesecake. (See the Recipes section for details!) Besides reducing the overall fat and sugar content, I lowered the sodium content, too.

Using my recipes can help you lose weight, lower and control your cholesterol and/or blood-sugar levels, and still allow you to enjoy delicious foods that deliver good nutrition and great "eye" appeal!

I didn't set out to impress anyone with fancy gourmet recipes that require unusual ingredients. Most of the mail I receive from people who've tried my recipes tells me that I made the right decision. They wanted (as my family and I did) to discover quick, tummy-pleasing, "common-folk" dishes that were healthy, too — and in my Healthy Exchanges recipes they found exactly what they were looking for.

My sister Jeanie is another good example of the Healthy Exchanges recipe user. She could probably best be described as a "noncooking" cook. If a recipe isn't easy, she doesn't want to be bothered, because she has more important things to do with her time. But she gladly takes the few minutes required to stir up her favorite Healthy Exchanges recipes!

The Four "Musts"

Before I included any recipe in this book, it had to meet my Four "Musts." I knew that if I didn't address these "Musts" from the very beginning, I would be just dieting, and only days or minutes away from falling off the "health wagon," as I call it — and into a binge where I would be keeping company again with cake donuts and hot fudge sundaes (my personal favorites . . . and downfalls!).

By eliminating unnecessary preparation and excess "bad" foods, I've made it much easier to live and eat healthily. Each of my recipes must be:

1. **Healthy.** Every recipe is low in sugar and fat and within a reasonable range for sodium. And because it is all of these, it is also low in calories and cholesterol. The prepared food can be eaten with confidence by diabetics and heart patients as well as anyone interested in losing weight or maintaining a weight loss.

2. **Easy to make.** Most people don't have the time or the inclination for complicated recipes. They just want to prepare something quickly and get it on the table as fast as possible. But they still want their families to be smiling when they leave the table. Simply put, they want dishes that are quick and easy to prepare — but that don't look like it!

3. **As tasty and good as they look.** If the foods we eat don't look, taste, smell, and feel like the family favorites we are used to eating, we won't be willing to eat them week in and week out.

We are all creatures of habit. If we grew up eating fried chicken with mashed potatoes every Sunday at noon, we may try poached chicken with plain potatoes once — but we'll go running back to our favorite greasy chicken as soon as we can get our hands on some. However, if we could enjoy healthy yet delicious oven-fried chicken with healthy yet satisfying mashed potatoes topped with rich, thick, healthy gravy, we would probably agree to give up the deep-fried chicken dinner. Rather than demanding we give up a beloved comfort food but instead serving a healthy version with all the great flavor of the original dish we remember, we can feel satisfied — and willing to make this "Healthy Exchange" for the rest of our lives.

Here's another example. "Good enough" will never be good enough for me again. My food has to be garnished in easy yet attractive ways so I feed my eyes as well as my stomach. That's why I sprinkle two tablespoons of chopped pecans on top of my **Cherry Dessert Pizza** (see recipe, page 367). This dish serves eight, which works out to about ³/₄ teaspoon of nuts per person. But we definitely taste that crunch as we enjoy that piece of dessert. And those delectable bites of

44

pecan help keep us from gobbling handfuls of nuts while watching TV. It's when we think we can't have something that we *dwell* on it constantly until we do get it. Moderation is the cornerstone of Healthy Exchanges recipes. My recipes include tiny amounts of mini chocolate chips, coconut, miniature marshmallows, nuts, and other foods I like to call "real-people" foods — not so-called "diet" food. This is just one of the distinctions that sets my cookbook apart from others that emphasize low-fat and/or low-sugar foods.

4. **Made from ingredients found in DeWitt, Iowa.** If the ingredients can be found in a small town with a population of 4,500 in the middle of an Iowa cornfield, then anyone ought to be able to find them, no matter where they shop! To make these recipes, you do not have to drive to a specialty store in a large city, or visit a health-food store in search of special ingredients.

Making It Quick, Easy, and More . . .

Once a recipe passes the Four Musts, I have a few additional requirements. One includes using the entire can if the container has to be opened with a can opener. The reason for this is simple: Only a few people are perfect Suzy and Homer Homemakers; most people are like me. If a recipe called for ⅓ cup tomato sauce, I would put the rest in the refrigerator with good intentions to use it up within a day or two — and six weeks later would probably have to toss it out because it was covered with moldy globs of green stuff. When I create a recipe, I devise a way to use the entire can and still have the dish taste delicious (and add up right when it comes to the mathematics of the exchanges for each serving).

Another test is what I call "Will It Play in Anytown, USA?" I ask myself if the retired person living on a meager pension or the young homemaker living on a modest paycheck can afford to prepare the recipe taking into account both equipment and ingredients. I ask myself if the person with arthritic hands or the parent with two small children underfoot can physically manage to make the recipe. If the answers are yes, that recipe will be included in my cookbooks or newsletters.

It's important to me that my recipes are simple to follow and to make.

Here are some of the ways I do this:

- I provide both the weight and the closest cup or spoon measurement for each ingredient. Why? Well, everyone who follows the major diet plans or uses the American Diabetic Association program is required to use a kitchen scale every day. But I know that in the real world this just won't happen. People say they're too busy to pull the scale out of the cupboard. Or they'd rather not use the measuring bowl and have to wash it. So my recipe says that 3 ounces of shredded reduced-fat cheese is equivalent to ³/₄ cup. I've measured this so often to make sure it's right. Why should you have to as well?

- I measure the final product and give the closest cup measurement per serving for anything that can't be cut into exact portions. For example, in a soup recipe, the serving size might be 1¹/₂ cups.

- I suggest baking all casseroles in an 8-by-8-inch pan for ease of portion control. If the dish serves four, just cut it down the center, turn the pan, and cut it down the center again. Each cut square yields one serving. Many cookbooks call for a 1¹/₂-quart casserole, but I find that most people tend to scoop out too much or too little while the rest of the casserole collapses into the center. There's no guesswork my way — just an easy and accurate means of managing portion size.

Measuring Success One Exchange at a Time

Healthy Exchanges recipes are unique for another reason: they provide nutritional information calculated in three ways.

1. **Diabetic Exchanges.** A Registered Dietitian has calculated the Diabetic Exchanges to conform to the guidelines established by

the American Diabetic Association. That makes this book a wonderful resource for diabetics, for those who need to cook for diabetic family members, and for professionals who educate diabetics about how to eat healthfully and control their condition.

2. *Calories, Fat Grams, and Fiber.* I list the fat grams right next to the calories. In traditional recipes, fat grams usually appear in the middle of the nutrient information. Now, if a person chooses to count fat grams or compare the percentage of fat calories to total calories, the information is quickly found. I also include fiber grams so you can monitor your fiber intake if you choose to.

3. *Weight Loss Choices®/Exchanges.* The recipes can be used by anyone attending the national weight-loss programs or support groups that count daily food intake by exchanges or selections instead of calories. (For a complete explanation of Healthy Exchanges Weight Loss Choices®/Exchanges, please refer to *The Healthy Exchanges Cookbook*.)

I've provided these three different kinds of nutritional measurements to make it easier for anyone and everyone to use my recipes as part of their commitment to a healthy lifestyle. I will do just about anything to make cooking healthier and easier for people — except wash their dishes!

Is Healthy Exchanges for You?

Are You Diabetic?
Do You Have Hypoglycemia?

My recipes are always low in sugar. A typical serving of lemon pie prepared in the traditional way provides approximately 500 calories with 30 grams of fat per serving, because processed sugar is the primary ingredient and fat not too far behind. My recipe for **Scrumptious Surprise Lemon Pie** is (see recipe, page 390) *208 calories per serving* with only 7 grams of fat and *no* added sugar! But just because I banished excess fats and sugars doesn't mean I've sacrificed any flavor. Besides, my pie can be cut into 8 pieces instead of the usual 12 servings per pie suggested in many diet recipes. (Did you know that one-sixth of a pie used to be the standard-size serving? Now, too many recipes expect you to settle for one-twelfth of a pie. But that skinny sliver leaves you hungry and going back for another piece. You're back to one-sixth of the pie again — and that might leave your tummy groaning and over-stuffed. But one-eighth of a pie is a satisfying, refreshing serving that will leave your palate happy!)

With Healthy Exchanges, diabetic and hypoglycemic patients can find the "real-world" food, especially desserts, they've been missing. You see, while my own blood sugar is normal, both my parents and two uncles developed adult-onset diabetes. So creating delicious low-sugar recipes is a priority for me.

Are You a Heart Disease Patient? Or Do You Just Need to Lower or Limit Cholesterol?

My Healthy Exchanges recipes are all low in fat, just right for you if you're recovering from a heart attack or if improving your cholesterol count is your goal. I have a recipe for **Crazy Pizza** (see recipe, page 323) which calls for real ingredients (*not* dietetic) and contains only 215 calories with 7 grams of fat per serving. It tastes just as good as a traditional recipe that delivers three times the amount of fat and almost twice the calories. And I don't skimp on the serving size! My approach provides a real savings in calories and fat without sacrificing flavor. While my own blood pressure and cholesterol are both within normal range, I know how important it is to stick to a diet low in fat. My parents both died of heart complications, so I've always been concerned about fat intake. This program provides dozens of delicious low-fat recipes to help you reach the best health possible.

Do You Want to Lose Weight — and Keep It Off for Good?

I am living proof that you can lose weight while eating dishes prepared from Healthy Exchanges recipes. I went from a much-too-tight size 28 to a healthy size 12 to 14 when I began eating my own creations. I always make sure the bases are covered when it comes to meeting nutritional needs, and *then* I throw in tiny amounts of delicious treats — foods like mini chocolate chips that are usually considered a "no-no" in traditional diet recipes. Yes, we can get by without these little touches, but do we want to? Should we have to?

When I was a "professional" dieter, a typical lunch would consist of a couple of slices of diet bread, tuna packed in water, diet mayonnaise, lettuce, a glass of skim milk, and a small apple. Good healthy choices, all of them. But why was I always reaching for a candy bar or cake donuts just an hour later? Because I had fed only my stomach, and not my heart, my eyes, or my soul. It was only when I began to enjoy a healthy piece of a real dessert every day that I began to lose weight and keep it off permanently. When I finally said NO to diets, I said YES to lasting weight loss!

The cardinal sin most people commit when going on a diet is preparing two different meals — skimpy get-the-weight-off-as-fast-as-possible food for the dieter, and real food for the rest of the family. My recipes can be eaten with confidence by anyone who wants to lose weight, but they are so tasty the entire family will gladly eat the same food. (I call it passing the "Cliff Lund Taste Test"!) When you cook with Healthy Exchanges, the burden of preparing two separate meals, not to mention the temptation of "sampling" the good stuff to be sure "it tastes right," has been eliminated. Now instead of short-term dieting and weight loss that never seems to last, you can take a step forward to healthy living for a lifetime!

Are You Simply Interested in Preventing Medical Problems from Developing? Are You Ready to Make a Commitment to Eat Healthier?

Maybe you're lucky enough to have no immediate medical concerns, but you would like to keep from developing them in the future. Perhaps you've seen all too clearly what the burdens of compromised health caused by a poor diet can be. You don't want to inherit the same "complications" you may have observed in parents and older family members, and you're determined to do your best to avoid future health problems by taking the necessary steps now. Healthy Exchanges will help you ensure lifelong good health.

Are You Interested in Quick and Easy Recipes the Entire Family Will Love?

Maybe you don't really care if a recipe is healthy or not. Maybe you have other priorities right now in your life, and you don't want to spend any more time than necessary in the kitchen. But because you and your family have to eat, you want a collection of good-tasting dishes that can be "thrown together" without much fuss. I will give you recipes for healthy, delicious food that often can be prepared in five minutes or less. (Not including unattended cooking time, but that time is freed for other projects!)

Did you answer "yes" to any of the questions on the past few pages? If you did, then **Healthy Exchanges** will give you just what you need — and deliciously, too!

Healthy Exchanges recipes have made a real difference in the lives of diabetics all over the country. You don't have to take my word for it, either. Here are excerpts from a few of their letters to me: From a young mother with diabetes who uses an insulin pump: "I've been a diabetic for 12 years and count carbohydrates in order to figure my insulin dosages. I use the carbohydrate counts more than the diabetic exchanges, but I'm glad to have both." (She told me she is looking forward to getting pregnant with a second child, especially since she won't have to exist on boring

snacks and meals again, as she did in her first pregnancy.) "I used to pack a cooler every day for work with all my little items to eat for snacks and meals throughout the day. I needed to eat six meals a day to obtain a nice level and low blood sugar. I used to eat the same thing every day. It'll be easier the second time with JoAnna's recipes."
— A.H., Illinois.

Another lady wrote, "My husband is not only diabetic, he had a bypass surgery last December, so you can see that we have to change a lot of old habits to improve our health and keep it that way. I really like the recipes using foods that we used to use before we started falling apart as we reached our sixties. Thanks for the help I've been wanting and not finding in other cookbooks!"
— M.R., Iowa.

Can eating the Healthy Exchanges way really make a difference in how your diabetes affects you? I was pleased to hear that it can. "My niece gave me your newsletter as a gift after my husband had a heart attack last July," wrote L.S. from Louisiana. "It has been the most-looked-forward-to piece of mail we get. It hasn't only benefited him but me as well. I have diabetes and have dropped my medication in half with the use of your recipes. They have really helped."

It means a lot to me to know that my recipes are helping people enjoy their lives to the fullest. A.P. from Arizona wrote, "I was recently diagnosed with diabetes and have been following a

54

closely prescribed program but find the inclusion of your unique recipes a great treat. 'Hats off' to you, JoAnna, for your creative talents and for sharing them with so many."

This last letter, sent to me by L.B. of Iowa, really touched my heart, because I will never forget how much my parents lost their pleasure in eating after they developed adult-onset diabetes.

"My husband is a diabetic of forty years, and trying to get him to eat right has always been a challenge. For most of those forty years eating low-sugar, low-fat foods was not only not very tasty, it just wasn't enjoyable. But boy have you made a change. My husband loves the food and it doesn't take me half a day to prepare it. You have made a wonderful change for the better in my husband's life. Keep up the marvelous work!"

A Few Rules for Success

A very important part of any journey is knowing where you are going and the best way to get there. If you plan and prepare before you start to cook, you should reach mealtime with foods to write home about!

1. **Read the entire recipe from start to finish** and be sure you understand the process involved. Check that you have all the equipment you will need *before* you begin.

2. **Check the ingredient list** and be sure you have *everything* and in the amounts required. Keep cooking sprays handy — while they're not listed as ingredients, I use them all the time (just a quick squirt!).

3. **Set out *all* the ingredients and equipment needed** to prepare the recipe on the counter near you *before* you start. Remember that old saying, *A stitch in time saves nine.* It applies in the kitchen, too.

4. **Do as much advance preparation as possible** before actually cooking. Chop, cut, grate, or whatever is needed to prepare the ingredients and have them ready before you start to mix. Turn the oven on at least ten

minutes before putting food in to bake, to allow the oven to preheat to the proper temperature.

5. **Use a kitchen timer** to tell you when the cooking or baking time is up. Because stove temperatures vary slightly by manufacturer, you may want to set your timer for five minutes less than the suggested time just to prevent overcooking. Check the progress of your dish at that time, then decide if you need the additional minutes or not.

6. **Measure carefully.** Use glass measures for liquids and metal or plastic cups for dry ingredients. My recipes are based on standard measurements. Unless I tell you it's a scant or full cup, measure the cup level.

7. **For best results, follow the recipe instructions exactly.** Feel free to substitute ingredients that *don't tamper* with the basic chemistry of the recipe, but be sure to leave key ingredients alone. For example, you could substitute sugar-free instant chocolate pudding for sugar-free butterscotch instant pudding, but if you use a six-serving package when a four-serving package is listed in the ingredients, or you use instant when cook-and-serve is required, you won't get the right result.

8. **Clean up as you go.** It is much easier to wash a few items at a time than to face a

whole counter of dirty dishes later. The same is true for spills on the counter or floor.

9. **Be careful about doubling or halving a recipe.** Though many recipes can be altered successfully to serve more or fewer people, *many cannot.* This is especially true when it comes to spices and liquids. If you try to double a recipe that calls for 1 teaspoon of pumpkin-pie spice, for example, and you double the spice, you may end up with a too-spicy taste. I usually suggest increasing spices or liquid by 1½ times when doubling a recipe. If it tastes a little bland to you, you can increase the spice to 1¾ times the original amount the next time you prepare the dish. Remember: You can always add more, but you can't take it out after it's stirred in.

The same is true with liquid ingredients. If you wanted to triple a recipe like my **Family Reunion Porkburgers** (see recipe, page 310) because you were planning to serve a crowd, you might think you should use three times as much of every ingredient. Don't, or you could end up with Porkburger Soup! The original recipe calls for 1¾ cups of chunky tomato sauce, so I'd suggest using 3½ cups of sauce when you *triple* the recipe (or 2¾ cups if you *double* it). You'll still have a good-tasting dish that won't run all over the plate.

10. **Write your reactions next to each recipe once you've served it.**

Yes, that's right, I'm giving you permission to write in this book. It's yours, after all. Ask yourself: Did everyone like it? Did you have to add another half teaspoon of chili seasoning to please your family, who like to live on the spicier side of the street? You may even want to rate the recipe on a scale of one to four stars (☆), depending on what you thought of it. (Four stars would be the top rating — and I hope you'll feel that way about many of my recipes.) Jotting down your comments while they are fresh in your mind will help you personalize the recipe to your own taste the next time you prepare it.

How to Read a Healthy Exchanges® Recipe

The Healthy Exchanges Nutritional Analysis

Before using these recipes, you may wish to consult your physician or health-care provider to be sure they are appropriate for you. The information in this book is not intended to take the place of any medical advice. It reflects my experiences, studies, research, and opinions regarding healthy eating.

Each recipe includes nutritional information calculated in three ways:
Diabetic exchanges
Calories, fiber, and fat grams
Healthy Exchanges Weight-Loss Choices®

or Exchanges (HE)

In every Healthy Exchanges recipe, the diabetic exchanges have been calculated by a registered dietitian. All the other calculations were done by computer, using the Food Processor II software. When the ingredient listing gives more than one choice, the first ingredient listed is the one used in the recipe analysis. Due to inevitable variations in the ingredients you choose to use, the nutritional values should be considered approximate.

The annotation "(limited)" following Protein counts in some recipes indicates that consumption of whole eggs should be limited to four per week.

Please note the following symbols:

☆ This star means read the recipe's directions carefully for special instructions about *division of ingredients*.

✳ This symbol indicates *freezes well*.

Exchange Lists

Exchange Lists are the "heart and soul" of the diabetic diet. Your doctor and/or dietitian will help you determine the number and kind of exchanges you should use for your meals and snacks. So many variables, such as your age, your sex, how active you are, and whether you need to lose weight are considered when determining what is best for you. While the exchange lists are designed primarily for people with diabetes and others who must follow special diets, this information really just makes good nutrition sense.

In order to help you incorporate my Healthy Exchanges recipes with your exchange requirements, I've included the American Diabetic Association's Exchange Lists in the following pages, provided to Healthy Exchanges by the ADA. The Diabetic Exchanges in Healthy Exchanges recipes are calculated by a registered dietitian using these lists so that you can make these delicious, commonsense healthy recipes a regular part of your diabetic eating plan.

The Exchange Lists are the basis of a meal-planning system designed by a committee of the American Diabetes Association and The American Dietetic Association. While designed primarily for people with diabetes and others who must follow special diets, the Exchange Lists are based on principles of good nutrition that apply to everyone. ©1995 American Diabetes Association, Inc., The American Dietetic Association.

Exchange Lists for Meal Planning

What Are Exchange Lists?

Exchange Lists are foods listed together because they are alike. Each serving of a food has about the same amount of carbohydrate, protein, fat, and calories as the other foods on that list. That is why any food on a list can be "exchanged" or traded for any other food on the same list. For example, you can trade the slice of bread you might eat for breakfast for one-half cup of cooked cereal. Each of these foods equals one *starch* choice.

Exchange Lists

Foods are listed with their serving sizes, which are usually measured after cooking. When you begin, you should measure the size of each serving. This may help you learn to "eyeball" correct serving sizes.

Common Measurements

3 tsp = 1 Tbsp	4 ounces = ½ cup
4 Tbsp = ¼ cup	8 ounces = 1 cup
5⅓ Tbsp = ⅓ cup	1 cup = ½ pint

The following chart shows the amount of nutrients in one serving from each list:

Groups/ Lists	Carbohydrates (grams)	Protein (grams)	Fat (grams)	Calories
Carbohydrate Group				
Starch	15	3	1 or less	80
Fruit	15	—	—	60
Milk				
Skim	12	8	0–3	90
Low-fat	12	8	5	120
Whole	12	8	8	150
Other carbohydrates	15	varies	varies	varies
Vegetables	5	2	—	25
Meat and Meat Substitute Group				
Very lean	—	7	0-1	35
Lean	—	7	3	55
Medium-fat	—	7	5	75
High-fat	—	7	8	100
Fat Group	—	—	5	45

The Exchange Lists provide you with a lot of food choices (foods from the basic food groups, foods with added sugars, free foods). This gives you variety in your meals. Several foods, such as dried beans and peas, bacon, and peanut butter, are on two lists. This gives you flexibility in putting your meals together. Whenever you choose new foods or vary your meal plan, monitor your blood glucose to see how these different foods affect your blood-glucose level.

Most foods in the Carbohydrate Group have about the same amount of carbohydrate per serving. You can exchange starch, fruit, or milk choices in your meal plan. Vegetables are in this group but contain only about 5 grams of carbohydrate.

A Word About Food Labels

Exchange information is based on food found in grocery stores. However, food companies often change the ingredients in their products. That is why you need to check the Nutrition Facts panel of the food label.

The Nutrition Facts tell you the number of calories and grams of carbohydrate, protein, and fat in one serving. Compare these numbers with the exchange information in this book to see how many exchanges you will be eating. In this way, food labels can help you add foods to your meal plans.

Ask your dietitian to help you use food label information to plan your meals.

Starch List

Cereals, grains, pasta, breads, crackers, snacks, starchy vegetables, and cooked dried beans, peas, and lentils are starches. In general, one starch is:

- ½ cup of cereal, grain, pasta, or starchy vegetable
- 1 ounce of a bread product, such as 1 slice of bread
- ¾ to 1 ounce of most snack foods. (Some snack foods may also have added fat.)

Nutrition Tips

1. Most starch choices are good sources of B vitamins.

2. Foods made from whole grains are good sources of fiber.

3. Dried beans and peas are a good source of protein and fiber.

Selection Tips

1. Choose starches made with little fat as often as you can.

2. Starchy vegetables prepared with fat count as one starch and one fat.

3. Bagels or muffins can be 2, 3, or 4 ounces in size and can, therefore, count as two, three, or four starch choices. Check the size you eat.

4. Dried beans, peas, and lentils are also found on the Meat and Meat Substitutes List.

5. Regular potato chips and tortilla chips are found on the Other Carbohydrates List.

6. Most of the serving sizes are measured after cooking.

7. Always check Nutrition Facts on the food label.

**One starch exchange equals
15 grams carbohydrate,
3 grams protein,
0–1 grams fat, and
80 calories.**

Bread

Bagel	$^1/_2$ (1 oz)
Bread, reduced calorie	2 slices (1$^1/_2$ oz)
Bread, white, whole wheat, pumpernickel, rye	1 slice (1 oz)
Bread sticks, crisp, 4 in. long X $^1/_2$ in.	2 ($^2/_3$ oz)
English muffin	$^1/_2$
Hot dog or hamburger bun	$^1/_2$ (1 oz)
Pita, 6 in. across	$^1/_2$
Raisin bread, unfrosted	1 slice (1 oz)
Roll, plain, small	1 (1 oz)
Tortilla, corn, 6 in. across	1
Tortilla, flour, 7–8 in. across	1
Waffle, 4$^1/_2$ in. square, reduced-fat	1

Cereals and Grains

Bran cereals	$\frac{1}{2}$ cup
Bulgur	$\frac{1}{2}$ cup
Cereals	$\frac{1}{2}$ cup
Cereals, unsweetened, ready to eat	$\frac{3}{4}$ cup
Cornmeal (dry)	3 Tbsp
Couscous	$\frac{1}{3}$ cup
Flour (dry)	3 Tbsp
Granola, low-fat	$\frac{1}{4}$ cup
Grape-Nuts	$\frac{1}{4}$ cup
Grits	$\frac{1}{2}$ cup
Kasha	$\frac{1}{2}$ cup
Millet	$\frac{1}{4}$ cup
Muesli	$\frac{1}{4}$ cup
Oats	$\frac{1}{2}$ cup
Pasta	$\frac{1}{2}$ cup
Puffed cereal	$1\frac{1}{2}$ cups
Rice milk	$\frac{1}{2}$ cup
Rice, white or brown	$\frac{1}{3}$ cup
Shredded Wheat	$\frac{1}{2}$ cup
Sugar-frosted cereal	$\frac{1}{2}$ cup
Wheat germ	3 Tbsp

Starchy Vegetables

Baked beans	$1/3$ cup
Corn	$1/2$ cup
Corn on cob, medium	1 (5 oz)
Mixed vegetables with corn, peas, or pasta	1 cup
Peas, green	$1/2$ cup
Plantain	$1/2$ cup
Potato, baked or boiled	1 small (3 oz)
Potato, mashed	$1/2$ cup
Squash, winter (acorn or butternut)	1 cup
Yam, sweet potato, plain	$1/2$ cup

Crackers and Snacks

Animal crackers	8
Graham crackers, $2^{1}/_{2}$ in. square	3
Matzoh	$3/4$ oz
Melba toast	4 slices
Oyster crackers	24
Popcorn (popped, no fat added or low-fat microwave)	3 cups
Pretzels	$3/4$ oz

Rice cakes, 4 in. across	2
Saltine-type crackers	6
Snack chips, fat–free (tortilla, potato)	15–20 (³/₄ oz)
Whole-wheat crackers, no fat added	2–5 (³/₄ oz)

Dried Beans, Peas, and Lentils
(Count as 1 starch exchange, plus 1 very lean meat exchange.)

Beans and peas (garbanzo, pinto, kidney, white, split, black-eyed)	¹/₂ cup
Lima beans	²/₃ cup
Lentils	¹/₂ cup
Miso △	3 Tbsp

Starchy Foods Prepared with Fat
(Count as 1 starch exchange, plus 1 fat exchange.)

Biscuit, 2¹/₂ in. across	1
Chow mein noodles	¹/₂ cup
Corn bread, 2 in. cube	1 (2 oz)
Crackers, round butter type	6
Croutons	1 cup

△ = 400 mg or more of sodium per serving

French-fried potatoes	16–25 (3 oz)
Granola	$\frac{1}{4}$ cup
Muffin, small	1 (1$\frac{1}{2}$ oz)
Pancake, 4 in. across	2
Popcorn, microwave	3 cups
Sandwich crackers, cheese or peanut-butter filling	3
Stuffing, bread (prepared)	$\frac{1}{2}$ cup
Taco shell, 6 in. across	2
Waffle, 4$\frac{1}{2}$ in. square	1
Whole-wheat crackers, fat added	4–6 (1 oz)

Some food you buy uncooked will weigh less after you cook it. Starches often swell in cooking, so a small amount of uncooked starch will become a much larger amount of cooked food. The following table shows some of the changes:

Food (Starch Group)	Uncooked	Cooked
Oatmeal	3 Tbsp	$\frac{1}{2}$ cup
Cream of Wheat	2 Tbsp	$\frac{1}{2}$ cup
Grits	3 Tbsp	$\frac{1}{2}$ cup
Rice	2 Tbsp	$\frac{1}{3}$ cup
Spaghetti	$\frac{1}{4}$ cup	$\frac{1}{2}$ cup

Noodles	⅓ cup	½ cup
Macaroni	¼ cup	½ cup
Dried beans	¼ cup	½ cup
Dried peas	¼ cup	½ cup
Lentils	3 Tbsp	½ cup

Fruit List

Fresh, frozen, canned, and dried fruits and fruit juices are on this list. In general, one fruit exchange is:

- 1 small to medium fresh fruit
- ½ cup of canned or fresh fruit or fruit juice
- ¼ cup of dried fruit.

Nutrition Tips
1. Fresh, frozen, and dried fruits have about 2 grams of fiber per choice. Fruit juices contain very little fiber.
2. Citrus fruits, berries, and melons are good sources of vitamin C.

Selection Tips
1. Count ½ cup cranberries or rhubarb sweetened with sugar substitutes as free foods.
2. Read the Nutrition Facts on the food label. If one serving has more than 15 grams carbohydrate, you will need to adjust the size of the serving you eat or drink.

3. Portion sizes for canned fruits are for the fruit and a small amount of juice.

4. Whole fruit is more filling than fruit juice and may be a better choice.

5. Food labels for fruits may contain the words "no sugar added" or "unsweetened." This means that no sucrose (table sugar) has been added.

6. Generally, fruit canned in extralight syrup has the same amount of carbohydrate per serving as the "no sugar added" or the juice pack. All canned fruits on the Fruit List are based on one of these three types of pack.

**One fruit exchange equals
15 grams carbohydrate and
60 calories.
The weight includes skin,
core, seeds, and rind.**

Fruit

Apple, unpeeled, small	1 (4 oz)
Applesauce, unsweetened	½ cup
Apples, dried	4 rings
Apricots, fresh	4 whole (5½ oz)
Apricots, dried	8 halves
Apricots, canned	½ cup

Banana, small	1 (4 oz)
Blackberries	³/₄ cup
Blueberries	³/₄ cup
Cantaloupe, small	¹/₃ melon (11 oz) or 1 cup cubes
Cherries, sweet, fresh	12 (3 oz)
Cherries, sweet, canned	¹/₂ cup
Dates	3
Figs, fresh	1¹/₂ large or 2 medium (3¹/₂ oz)
Figs, dried	1¹/₂
Fruit cocktail	¹/₂ cup
Grapefruit, large	¹/₂ (11 oz)
Grapefruit sections, canned	³/₄ cup
Grapes, small	17 (3 oz)
Honeydew melon	1 slice (10 oz) or 1 cup cubes
Kiwi	1 (3¹/₂ oz)
Mandarin oranges, canned	³/₄ cup
Mango, small	¹/₂ fruit (5 oz) or ¹/₂ cup
Nectarine, small	1 (5 oz)
Orange, small	1 (6¹/₂ oz)
Papaya	¹/₂ fruit (8 oz) or 1 cup cubes

Peach, medium, fresh	1 (6 oz)
Peaches, canned	¹/₂ cup
Pear, large, fresh	¹/₂ (4 oz)
Pears, canned	¹/₂ cup
Pineapple, fresh	³/₄ cup
Pineapple, canned	¹/₂ cup
Plums, small	2 (5 oz)
Plums, canned	¹/₂ cup
Prunes, dried	3
Raisins	2 Tbsp
Raspberries	1 cup
Strawberries	1¹/₄ cup whole berries
Tangerines, small	2 (8 oz)
Watermelon	1 slice (13¹/₂ oz) or 1¹/₄ cup cubes

Fruit Juice

Apple juice/cider	¹/₂ cup
Cranberry juice cocktail	¹/₃ cup
Cranberry juice cocktail, reduced-calorie	1 cup
Fruit juice blends, 100% juice	¹/₃ cup

Grape juice	⅓ cup
Grapefruit juice	½ cup
Orange juice	½ cup
Pineapple juice	½ cup
Prune juice	⅓ cup

Milk List

Different types of milk and milk products are on this list. Cheeses are on the Meat List, and cream and other dairy fats are on the Fat List. Based on the amount of fat they contain, milks are divided into skim/very low fat milk, low-fat milk, and whole milk. One choice of these includes:

	Carbohydrates (grams)	Protein (grams)	Fat (grams)	Calories
Skim/very low fat	12	8	0-3	90
Low-fat	12	8	5	120
Whole	12	8	8	150

Nutrition Tips
1. Milk and yogurt are good sources of calcium and protein. Check the food label.

2. The higher the fat content of milk and yogurt, the greater the amount of saturated fat and cholesterol. Choose lower-fat varieties.

3. For those who are lactose intolerant, look for lactose-reduced or lactose-free varieties of milk.

Selection Tips

1. One cup equals 8 fluid ounces or $\frac{1}{2}$ pint.

2. Look for chocolate milk, frozen yogurt, and ice cream on the Other Carbohydrates List.

3. Nondairy creamers are on the Free Food List.

4. Look for rice milk on the Starch List.

5. Look for soy milk on the Medium-Fat Meat List.

One milk exchange equals 12 grams carbohydrate and 8 grams protein.

Skim and Very Low Fat Milk

Skim milk	1 cup
$\frac{1}{2}$% milk	1 cup
1% milk	1 cup
Nonfat or low-fat buttermilk	1 cup
Evaporated skim milk	$\frac{1}{2}$ cup

Nonfat dry milk	$^1/_3$ cup dry
Plain nonfat yogurt	$^3/_4$ cup
Nonfat or low-fat fruit-flavored yogurt sweetened with aspartame or a nonnutritive sweetener	1 cup

Low-Fat (5 grams fat per serving)

2% milk	1 cup
Plain low-fat yogurt	$^3/_4$ cup
Sweet acidophilus milk	1 cup

Whole Milk (8 grams fat per serving)

Whole milk	1 cup
Evaporated whole milk	$^1/_2$ cup
Goat's milk	1 cup
Kefir	1 cup

Other Carbohydrates List

You can substitute food choices from this list for a starch, fruit, or milk choice on your meal plan. Some choices will also count as one or more fat choices.

Nutrition Tips
1. These foods can be substituted in your meal

plan, even though they contain added sugars or fat. However, they do not contain as many important vitamins and minerals as the choices on the Starch, Fruit, or Milk lists.

2. When planning to include these foods in your meal, be sure to include foods from all the lists to eat a balanced meal.

Selection Tips

1. Because many of these foods are concentrated sources of carbohydrate and fat, the portion sizes are often very small.

2. Always check Nutrition Facts on the food label. It will be your most accurate source of information.

3. Many fat-free or reduced-fat products made with fat replacers contain carbohydrate. When eaten in large amounts, they may need to be counted. Talk with your dietitian to determine how to count these in your meal plan.

4. Look for fat-free salad dressings in smaller amounts on the Free Foods List.

**One exchange equals
15 grams carbohydrate, or 1 starch,
or 1 fruit, or 1 milk**

Food	Serving Size	Exchanges per Serving
Angel food cake, unfrosted	$^1/_{12}$ cake	2 carbohydrates
Brownie, small, unfrosted	2 in. square	1 carbohydrate, 1 fat
Cake, unfrosted	2 in. square	1 carbohydrate, 1 fat
Cake, frosted	2 in. square	2 carbohydrates, 1 fat
Cookie, fat-free	2 small	1 carbohydrate
Cookie or sandwich cookie with creme filling	2 small	1 carbohydrate, 1 fat
Cupcake, frosted	1 small	2 carbohydrates, 1 fat
Cranberry sauce, jellied	$^1/_4$ cup	2 carbohydrates
Doughnut, plain cake	1 medium ($1^1/_2$ oz)	$1^1/_2$ carbohydrates, 2 fats
Doughnut, glazed	$3^3/_4$ in. across (2 oz)	2 carbohydrates, 2 fats
Fruit juice bars, frozen, 100% juice	1 bar (3 oz)	1 carbohydrate
Fruit snacks, chewy (pureed fruit concentrate)	1 roll ($^3/_4$ oz)	1 carbohydrate
Fruit spreads, 100% fruit	1 Tbsp	1 carbohydrate
Gelatin, regular	$^1/_2$ cup	1 carbohydrate

Food	Serving Size	Exchanges per Serving
Ginger Snaps	3	1 carbohydrate
Granola bar	1 bar	1 carbohydrate, 1 fat
Granola bar, fat-free	1 bar	2 carbohydrates
Hummus	1/3 cup	1 carbohydrate, 1 fat
Ice cream	1/2 cup	1 carbohydrate, 2 fats
Ice cream, light	1/2 cup	1 carbohydrate, 1 fat
Ice cream, fat-free, no sugar added	1/2 cup	1 carbohydrate
Jam or jelly, regular	1 Tbsp	1 carbohydrate
Milk, chocolate, whole	1 cup	2 carbohydrates, 1 fat
Pie, fruit, two crusts	1/6 pie	3 carbohydrates, 2 fats
Pie, pumpkin or custard	1/8 pie	1 carbohydrate, 2 fats
Potato chips	12–18 (1 oz)	1 carbohydrate, 2 fats
Pudding, regular (made with low-fat milk)	1/2 cup	2 carbohydrates

Food	Serving Size	Exchanges per Serving
Pudding, sugar-free (made with low-fat milk)	½ cup	1 carbohydrate
Salad dressing, fat-free△	¼ cup	1 carbohydrate
Sherbet, sorbet	½ cup	2 carbohydrates
Spaghetti or pasta sauce, canned△	½ cup	1 carbohydrate, 1 fat
Sweet roll or Danish	1 (2½ oz)	2½ carbohydrates, 2 fats
Syrup, light	2 Tbsp	1 carbohydrate
Syrup, regular	1 Tbsp	1 carbohydrate
Syrup, regular	¼ cup	4 carbohydrates
Tortilla chips	6–12 (1 oz)	1 carbohydrate, 2 fats
Yogurt, frozen, low-fat, fat-free	⅓ cup	1 carbohydrate, 0–1 fat
Yogurt, frozen, fat-free, no sugar added	½ cup	1 carbohydrate
Yogurt, low-fat with fruit	1 cup	3 carbohydrates, 0–1 fat
Vanilla wafers	5	1 carbohydrate, 1 fat

△ = 400 mg or more sodium per exchange

Vegetable List

Vegetables that contain small amounts of carbohydrates and calories are on this list. Vegetables contain important nutrients. Try to eat at least two or three vegetable choices each day. In general, one vegetable exchange is:

- ½ cup of cooked vegetables or vegetable juice
- 1 cup of raw vegetables

If you eat one to two vegetable choices at a meal or snack, you do not have to count the calories or carbohydrates because they contain small amounts of these nutrients.

Nutrition Tips

1. Fresh and frozen vegetables have less added salt than canned vegetables. Drain and rinse canned vegetables if you want to remove some salt.

2. Choose more dark green and dark yellow vegetables, such as spinach, broccoli, romaine, carrots, chilis, and peppers.

3. Broccoli, brussels sprouts, cauliflower, greens, peppers, spinach, and tomatoes are good sources of vitamin C.

4. Vegetables contain 1 to 4 grams of fiber per serving.

Selection Tips

1. A 1-cup portion of broccoli is a portion about the size of a lightbulb.

2. Tomato sauce is different from spaghetti sauce, which is on the Other Carbohydrates List.

3. Canned vegetables and juices are available without added salt.

4. If you eat more than 4 cups of raw vegetables or 2 cups of cooked vegetables at one meal, count them as one carbohydrate choice.

5. Starchy vegetables, such as corn, peas, winter squash, and potatoes, that contain larger amounts of calories and carbohydrates are on the Starch List.

**One vegetable exchange equals
5 grams carbohydrates,
2 grams protein,
0 grams fat, and
25 calories.**

Vegetables

Artichoke
Artichoke hearts
Asparagus
Beans (green, wax,
    Italian)
Bean sprouts
Beets
Broccoli
Brussels sprouts
Cabbage
Carrots
Cauliflower
Celery
Cucumber
Eggplant
Green onions or
    scallions
Greens (collard,
    kale, mustard,
    turnip)
Kohlrabi
Leeks
Mixed vegetables
    (without corn,
    peas, or pasta)

Mushrooms
Okra
Onions
Pea pods
Peppers (all varieties)
Radishes
Salad greens (endive,
    escarole, lettuce,
    romaine, spinach)
Sauerkraut$^\triangle$
Spinach
Summer squash
Tomato
Tomatoes, canned
Tomato sauce$^\triangle$
Tomato/vegetable
    juice$^\triangle$
Turnips
Water chestnuts
Watercress
Zucchini

$\triangle$ = 400 mg or more sodium per exchange

Meat and Meat Substitutes List

Meat and meat substitutes that contain both protein and fat are on this list. In general, one meat exchange is:

- 1 oz meat, fish, poultry, or cheese,
- ½ cup dried beans.

Based on the amount of fat they contain, meats are divided into very lean, lean, medium-fat, and high-fat lists. This is done so you can see which ones contain the least amount of fat. One ounce (one exchange of each) of these includes:

	Carbohydrates (grams)	Protein (grams)	Fat (grams)	Calories
Very lean	0	7	0–1	35
Lean	0	7	3	55
Medium-fat	0	7	5	75
High-fat	0	7	8	100

Nutrition Tips

1. Choose very lean and lean meat choices whenever possible. Items from the high-fat group are high in saturated fat, cholesterol, and calories and can raise blood cholesterol levels.

2. Meats do not have any fiber.

3. Dried beans, peas, and lentils are good sources of fiber.

4. Some processed meats, seafood, and soy products may contain carbohydrate when consumed in large amounts. Check the Nutrition Facts on the label to see if the amount is close to 15 grams. If so, count it as a carbohydrate choice as well as a meat choice.

Selection Tips

1. Weigh meat after cooking and removing bones and fat. Four ounces of raw meat are equal to 3 ounces of cooked meat. Some examples of meat portions are:

   - 1 ounce cheese = one meat choice and is about the size of a 1-inch cube.

   - 2 ounces meat = two meat choices, such as 1 small chicken leg or thigh or ½ cup cottage cheese or tuna.

   - 3 ounces meat = three meat choices and are about the size of a deck of cards, such as 1 medium pork chop, 1 small hamburger, ½ of a whole chicken breast, 1 unbreaded fish fillet.

2. Limit your choices from the high-fat group to three times per week or less.

3. Most grocery stores stock Select and Choice grades of meat. Select grades of meat are the leanest meats. Choice grades contain a mod-

erate amount of fat, and Prime cuts of meat have the highest amount of fat. Restaurants usually serve Prime cuts of meat.

4. "Hamburger" may contain added seasoning and fat, but ground beef does not.

5. Read labels to find products that are low in fat and cholesterol (5 grams or less of fat per serving).

6. Dried beans, peas, and lentils are also found on the Starch List.

7. Peanut butter, in smaller amounts, is also found on the Fats List.

8. Bacon, in smaller amounts, is also found on the Fats List.

Meal Planning Tips

1. Bake, roast, broil, grill, poach, steam, or boil these foods rather than fry them.

2. Place meat on a rack so the fat will drain off during cooking.

3. Use a nonstick spray and a nonstick pan to brown or fry foods.

4. Trim off visible fat before or after cooking.

5. If you add flour, bread crumbs, coating mixes, fat, or marinades when cooking, ask your dietitian how to count these in your meal plan.

Very Lean Meat and Substitutes List

One exchange equals 0 grams carbohydrates, 7 grams protein, 0–1 grams fat, and 35 calories.

One very lean meat exchange is equal to any of the following items:

Poultry: Chicken or turkey (white meat, no skin), Cornish hen (no skin)   1 oz

Fish: Fresh or frozen cod, flounder, haddock, halibut, trout; tuna, fresh or canned in water   1 oz

Shellfish: Clams, crab, lobster, scallops, shrimp, imitation shellfish   1 oz

Game: Duck or pheasant (no skin), venison, buffalo, ostrich   1 oz

Cheese with 1 gram or less fat per ounce:
Nonfat or low-fat cottage cheese   ¼ cup
Fat-free cheese   1 oz

Other: Processed sandwich meats with 1 gram or less fat per ounce, such as deli thin, shaved meats, chipped beef,△ turkey, ham   1 oz

△ = 400 mg or more sodium per exchange

Egg whites	2
Egg substitutes, plain	¼ cup
Hot dogs with 1 gram of fat or less per ounce△	1 oz
Kidney (high in cholesterol)	1 oz
Sausage with 1 gram or less of fat per ounce	1 oz

Count as one very lean meat and one starch exchange:

Dried beans, peas, lentils, cooked	½ cup

Lean Meat and Substitutes List

One exchange equals 0 grams carbohydrate, 7 grams protein, 3 grams fat, and 55 calories.

One lean meat exchange is equal to any of the following items:

Beef: USDA Select or Choice grades of lean beef trimmed of fat, such as round, sirloin, and flank steak; tenderloin; roast (rib, chuck, rump); steak (T-bone, porterhouse, cubed), ground round   1 oz

△ = 400 mg or more sodium per exchange

Pork: Lean pork, such as fresh ham; canned, cured, or boiled ham; Canadian bacon△; tenderloin, center loin chop — 1 oz

Lamb: Roast, chop, leg — 1 oz

Veal: Lean chop, roast — 1 oz

Poultry: Chicken, turkey (dark meat, no skin), chicken white meat (with skin), domestic duck or goose (well drained of fat, no skin) — 1 oz

Fish: Herring (uncreamed or smoked) — 1 oz
  Oysters — 6 medium

  Salmon (fresh or canned), catfish — 1 oz
  Sardines (canned) — 2 medium

  Tuna (canned in oil, drained) — 1 oz

Game: Goose (no skin), rabbit — 1 oz

Cheese: 4.5% fat cottage cheese — ¼ cup
  Grated Parmesan — 2 Tbsp
  Cheeses with 3 grams or less fat per ounce — 1 oz

Other: Hot dogs with 3 grams or less of fat per ounce△ — 1½ oz
  Processed sandwich meat with 3 grams or less fat per ounce, such

△ = 400 mg or more sodium per exchange

as turkey, pastrami, or kielbasa   1 oz
Liver, heart (high in cholesterol)   1 oz

Medium-Fat Meat and Substitutes List

One exchange equals 0 grams carbohydrate, 7 grams protein, 5 grams fat, and 75 calories.

One medium-fat exchange is equal to any one of the following items:

Beef: Most beef products fall into this category (ground beef, meat loaf, corned beef, short ribs, Prime grades of meat trimmed of fat, such as prime rib)   1 oz

Pork: Top loin, chop, Boston butt, cutlet   1 oz

Lamb: Rib roast, ground   1 oz

Veal: Cutlet (ground or cubed, un-breaded)   1 oz

Poultry: Chicken dark meat (with skin), ground turkey or ground chicken, fried chicken (with skin)   1 oz

Fish: Any fried fish product   1 oz

Cheese: With 5 grams or less fat per ounce
Feta   1 oz
Mozzarella   1 oz
Ricotta   1 oz

Other:

Egg (high in cholesterol, limit to 3 per week)	1
Sausage with 5 grams or less of fat per ounce	1 oz
Soy milk	1 cup
Tempeh	¼ cup
Tofu	4 oz or ½ cup

High-Fat Meat and Substitutes List

One exchange equals 0 grams carbohydrate, 7 grams protein, 8 grams fat, and 100 calories.

Remember: These items are high in saturated fat, cholesterol, and calories and may raise blood cholesterol levels if eaten on a regular basis. One high-fat meat exchange is equal to any one of the following items:

Pork: Spareribs, ground pork, pork sausage	1 oz
Cheese: All regular cheeses, such as American,△ Cheddar, Monterey Jack, Swiss	1 oz
Other: Processed sandwich meats with 8 grams or less fat per ounce, such as bologna, pimiento loaf, salami	1 oz

△ = 400 mg or more sodium per exchange

Sausage, such as bratwurst, Italian, knockwurst, Polish, smoked	1 oz
Hot dog (turkey or chicken)△	1 (10/lb)
Bacon	3 slices (20/lb)

Count as one high-fat meat *plus* one fat exchange:

| Hot dog (beef, pork, or combination)△ | 1 (10/lb) |
| Peanut butter (contains saturated fat) | 2 Tbsp |

Fat List

Fats are divided into three groups, based on the main type of fat they contain: monounsaturated, polyunsaturated, and saturated. Small amounts of monounsaturated and polyunsaturated fats in the foods we eat are linked with good health benefits. Saturated fats are linked with heart disease and cancer. In general, one fat exchange is:

- 1 teaspoon regular margarine or vegetable oil
- 1 tablespoon of regular salad dressings.

△ = 400 mg or more sodium per exchange

Nutrition Tips

1. All fats are high in calories. Limit serving sizes for good nutrition and health.

2. Nuts and seeds contain small amounts of fiber, protein, and magnesium.

3. If blood pressure is a concern, choose fats in the unsalted form to help lower sodium intake, such as unsalted peanuts.

Serving Tips

1. Check the Nutrition Facts on food labels for serving sizes. One fat exchange is based on a serving size containing 5 grams of fat.

2. When selecting regular margarine, choose those with liquid vegetable oil as the first ingredient. Soft margarines are not as saturated as stick margarines. Soft margarines are healthier choices. Avoid those listing hydrogenated fat as the first ingredient.

3. When selecting low-fat margarines, look for liquid vegetable oil as the second ingredient. Water is usually the first ingredient.

4. When used in smaller amounts, bacon and peanut butter are counted as fat choices. When used in larger amounts, they are counted as high-fat meat choices.

5. Fat-free salad dressings are on the Other Carbohydrates List and the Free Foods List.

6. See the Free Foods List for nondairy coffee creamers, whipped topping, and fat-free

products, such as margarines, salad dressings, mayonnaise, sour cream, cream cheese, and nonstick cooking spray.

Monounsaturated Fats List

One fat exchange equals 5 grams fat and 45 calories.

Avocado, medium	⅛ (1 oz)
Oil (canola, olive, peanut)	1 tsp
Olives: ripe (black)	8 large
green (stuffed)△	10 large
Nuts	
almonds, cashews	6 nuts
mixed (50% peanuts)	6 nuts
peanuts	10 nuts
pecans	4 halves
Peanut butter, smooth or crunchy	2 tsp
Sesame seeds	1 Tbsp
Tahini paste	2 tsp

Polyunsaturated Fats List

One fat exchange equals 5 grams fat and 45 calories.

Margarine: stick, tub, squeeze	1 tsp
lower-fat	
(30% to 50% vegetable oil)	1 Tbsp
Mayonnaise: regular	1 tsp
reduced-fat	1 Tbsp
Nuts, walnuts, English	4 halves
Oil (corn, safflower, soybean)	1 tsp

△ = 400 mg or more sodium per exchange

Salad dressing: regular$^\triangle$	1 Tbsp
reduced-fat	2 Tbsp
Miracle Whip Salad Dressing®:	
regular	2 tsp
reduced-fat	1 Tbsp
Seeds: pumpkin, sunflower	1 Tbsp

Saturated Fats List [†]

One fat exchange equals 5 grams fat and 45 calories.

Bacon, cooked	1 slice (20 slices/lb)
Bacon grease	1 tsp
Butter: stick	1 tsp
whipped	2 tsp
reduced-fat	1 Tbsp
Chitterlings, boiled	2 Tbsp ($^1/_2$ oz)
Coconut, sweetened, shredded	2 Tbsp
Cream, half and half	2 Tbsp
Cream cheese: regular	1 Tbsp ($^1/_2$ oz)
reduced-fat	2 Tbsp (1 oz)
Fatback or salt pork, see below*	
Shortening or lard	1 tsp
Sour cream: regular	2 Tbsp
reduced-fat	3 Tbsp

$\triangle$ = 400 mg or more sodium per exchange
[†] Saturated fats can raise blood cholesterol levels.
* Use a piece 1 in. by 1 in. by ¼ in. if you plan to eat the fatback cooked with vegetables. Use a piece 2 in. by 1 in. by ½ in. when eating only the vegetables with the fatback removed.

Free Foods List

A free food is any food or drink that contains fewer than 20 calories or 5 grams of carbohydrate per serving. Food with a serving size listed should be limited to three servings per day. Be sure to spread them out throughout the day. Eating all three servings at one time could affect your blood-glucose level. Foods listed without a serving size can be eaten as often as you like.

Fat-Free or Reduced-Fat Foods

Cream cheese, fat-free	1 Tbsp
Creamers, nondairy, liquid	1 Tbsp
Creamers, nondairy, powdered	2 tsp
Mayonnaise, fat-free	1 Tbsp
Mayonnaise, reduced-fat	1 tsp
Margarine, fat-free	4 Tbsp
Margarine, reduced-fat	1 tsp
Miracle Whip®, nonfat	1 Tbsp
Miracle Whip®, reduced-fat	1 tsp
Nonstick cooking spray	
Salad dressing, fat-free	1 Tbsp
Salad dressing, fat-free, Italian	2 Tbsp
Salsa	¼ cup
Sour cream, fat-free, reduced-fat	1 Tbsp
Whipped topping, regular or light	2 Tbsp

Sugar-Free or Low-Sugar Foods

Candy, hard, sugar-free	1 candy
Gelatin dessert, sugar-free	
Gelatin, unflavored	

Gum, sugar-free
Jam or jelly, low-sugar or light   2 tsp
Sugar substitutes*
Syrup, sugar-free   2 Tbsp

Drinks
Bouillon, broth, consomme△
Bouillon or broth, low-sodium
Carbonated or mineral water
Cocoa powder, unsweetened
Coffee
Club soda
Diet soft drinks, sugar-free
Drink mixes, sugar-free
Tea
Tonic water, sugar-free

Condiments
Catsup
Horseradish
Lemon juice
Lime juice
Mustard

* Sugar substitutes, alternatives, or replacements that are approved by the Food and Drug Administration (FDA) are safe to use. Common brand names include:
     Equal® (aspartame)
     Sprinkle Sweet (saccharin)
     Sweet One (acesulfame K)
     Sweet-10 (saccharin)
     Sugar-Twin (saccharin)
     Sweet 'n Low (saccharin)

△ = 400 mg or more of sodium per choice

Pickles, dill△
Soy sauce, regular or light△
Taco sauce
Vinegar

Seasonings

Be careful with seasonings that contain sodium or are salts, such as garlic or celery salt and lemon pepper.

Flavoring extracts
Garlic
Herbs, fresh or dried
Pimiento
Spices
Tabasco® or hot pepper sauce
Wine, used in cooking
Worcestershire sauce

Now that you've read through the official Exchange Lists from the American Diabetic Association, you're just about ready to start eating! You'll find in the pages that follow dozens of satisfying, easy-to-fix Healthy Exchanges recipes that have already been carefully calculated to fit your doctor's or dietitian's recommendations for your diabetic diet.

But before you go on, I want to tell you how other family members may benefit from making Healthy Exchanges recipes part of a new family-wide commitment to better health.

△ = 400 mg or more of sodium per choice

Most people using this cookbook may choose to count the Diabetic Exchanges provided, but other members of your family may decide to use the Healthy Exchanges Weight Loss Choices information (the line called *HE*) to work toward regaining their health or losing weight. The basic exchanges — Protein, Fat, Bread, Fruit, Skim Milk, and Vegetables — will work for anyone who is following one of the national weight-loss programs. However, a few words of explanation about two other categories included in my Healthy Exchanges Weight Loss Choices might be helpful.

Optional Calories

Foods that do not fit into any other group but are used in moderation in recipes are included in Optional Calories. Foods that are counted in this way include sugar-free gelatin and puddings, fat-free mayonnaise and dressings, reduced-calorie whipped toppings, reduced-calorie syrups and jams, chocolate chips, coconut, and canned broth. Optional Calories should generally not exceed 150 calories per day.

Sliders™

These are 80 Optional Calorie increments that do not fit into any particular category. You can choose which food group to *slide* it into. It is wise to limit this selection to approximately three to four per day to ensure the best possible nutrition for your body while still enjoying an occasional treat.

Sliders (Sl) may be used in either of the following ways:

1. If you have consumed all of your Protein, Bread, Fruit, or Skim Milk Weight Loss Choices for the day, and you want to eat additional foods from those food groups, you simply use a Slider. It's what I call "healthy horse trading." Remember that Sliders may not be traded for choices in the Vegetables or Fats food groups.

2. Additional Sliders, if you choose to include them, may also be deducted from your Optional Calories (OC) for the day or week: ¼ Sl equals 20 OC; ½ Sl equals 40 OC; ¾ Sl equals 60 OC; and 1 Sl equals 80 OC. This way, you can choose the food group to *slide* it into.

If you would like more information about the Healthy Exchanges Weight Loss Choices eating plan, please consult *Healthy Exchanges Cookbook* or *HELP: Healthy Exchanges Lifetime Plan.*

Advice About Sodium, Fats, and Processed Foods

Sodium

Most people consume more sodium than their bodies need. The American Diabetes Association and the American Heart Association recommend limiting daily sodium intake to no more than 3,000 milligrams per day. If your doctor suggests you limit your sodium even more, then *you really must read labels*.

Sodium is an essential nutrient and should not be completely eliminated. It helps to regulate blood volume and is needed for normal daily muscle and nerve functions. Most of us, however, have no trouble getting "all we need" and then some.

As with everything else, moderation is my approach. I rarely ever have salt on my list as an added ingredient. But if you're especially sodium sensitive, make the right choices for you — and save high-sodium foods such as sauerkraut for an occasional treat.

I use lots of spices to enhance flavors, so you won't notice the absence of salt. In the few cases where it is used, it's vital for the success of the recipe, so please don't omit it.

When I do use an ingredient high in sodium, I try to compensate by using low-sodium products in the remainder of the recipe. Many fat-free products are a little higher in sodium to make up for any loss of flavor that disappeared along with the fat. But when I take advantage of these fat-free, higher-sodium products, I stretch that ingredient within the recipe, lowering the amount of sodium per serving. A good example is my use of fat-free canned soups. While the suggested number of servings per can is two, I make sure my final creation serves at least four and sometimes six. So the soup's sodium has been "watered down" from one-third to one-half of the original amount.

Even if you don't have to watch your sodium intake for medical reasons, using moderation is another "healthy exchange" to make on your own journey to good health.

Fat Percentages

We've been told that 30 percent is the magic number — that we should limit fat intake to 30 percent or less of our total calories. It's good advice, and I try to have a weekly average of 15 to 25 percent myself. I believe any less than 15 percent is really just another restrictive diet that won't last. And more than 25 percent on a regular basis is too much of a good thing.

When I started listing fat grams along with calories in my recipes, I was tempted to include the percentage of calories from fat. After all, in the vast majority of my recipes, that percentage is well below 30 percent. This even includes my pie recipes that allow you a realistic serving instead of many "diet" recipes that tell you a serving is one-twelfth of a pie.

Figuring fat grams is easy enough. Each gram of fat equals 9 calories. Multiply fat grams by 9, then divide that number by the total calories to get the percentage of calories from fat.

So why don't I do it? After consulting four registered dietitians for advice, I decided to omit this information. They felt that it's too easy for people to become obsessed by that 30 percent figure, which is after all supposed to be a percentage of total calories over the course of a day or a week. We mustn't feel we can't include a healthy ingredient such as pecans or olives in one recipe just because, on its own, it has more than 30 percent of its calories from fat.

An example of this would be a casserole made with 90 percent lean red meat. Most of us benefit from eating red meat in moderation, as it provides iron and niacin in our diets, and it also makes life more enjoyable for us and those who eat with us. If we *only* look at the percentage of calories from fat in a serving of this one dish, which might be as high as 40 to 45 percent, we might choose not to include this recipe in our weekly food plan.

The dietitians suggested that it's important to consider the total picture when making such decisions. As long as your overall food plan keeps fat calories to 30 percent, it's all right to enjoy an occasional dish that is somewhat higher in fat content. Healthy foods I include *in moderation* include 90 percent lean red meat, olives, and nuts. I don't eat these foods every day, and I know you don't either. But occasionally, in a good recipe, they make all the difference in the world between just getting by (deprivation) and truly enjoying your food.

Remember, the goal is eating in a healthy way so you can enjoy and live well the rest of your life.

Saturated Fats and Cholesterol

You'll see that I don't provide calculations for saturated fats or cholesterol amounts in my recipes. It's for the simple and yet not so simple reason that accurate, up-to-date, brand-specific information can be difficult to obtain from food manufacturers, especially since the way in which they produce food keeps changing rapidly. But once more I've consulted with registered dietitians and other professionals and found that because I use only a few products that are high in saturated fat, and use them in such limited quantities, my recipes are suitable for patients concerned about controlling or lowering cholesterol. You'll also find that whenever I do use one of these ingredients *in moderation,* everything else in the recipe, and in the meals my family and I enjoy, is low in fat.

Processed Foods

Some people have asked how "healthy" recipes can so often use "processed foods" — ready-made products like canned soups, prepared pie-crusts, frozen potatoes, and frozen whipped topping. Well, I believe that such foods, used properly (that word *moderation* again) as part of a healthy lifestyle, have a place as ingredients in healthy recipes.

I'm not in favor of spraying everything we eat with chemicals, and I don't mean that all our foods should come out of packages. But I do think we should use the best available products to make cooking easier and foods taste better. I take advantage of good low-fat and low-sugar products, and my recipes are created for busy people like me who want to eat well and eat healthfully. I don't expect people to visit out-of-the-way health food stores or find time to cook beans from scratch — because I don't. There are lots of very good processed foods available in your local grocery store, and they can make it so much easier to enjoy the benefits of healthy eating.

Most of us can't grow fresh food in the backyard, and many people don't even have a nearby farmer's market. But instead of saying, "Well, I can't get to the health food store so why not eat that hot fudge sundae?" you gotta play ball where your ball field is. I want to help you figure out ways to make living healthfully *doable* and *livable wherever you live,* or you're not going to stick with it.

My Best Healthy Exchanges Tips and Tidbits

Measurements, General Cooking Tips, and Basic Ingredients

The word **moderation** best describes **my use of fats, sugar substitutes,** and **sodium** in these recipes. Wherever possible, I've used cooking spray for sautéing and for browning meats and vegetables. I also use reduced-calorie margarine and no-fat mayonnaise and salad dressings. Lean ground turkey *or* ground beef can be used in the recipes. Just be sure whatever you choose is at least *90 percent lean.*

I've also included **small amounts of sugar and brown sugar substitutes as the sweetening agent** in many of the recipes. I don't drink a hundred cans of soda a day or eat enough artificially sweetened foods in a twenty-four-hour period to be troubled by sugar substitutes. But if this is a concern of yours and you *do not* need to watch your sugar intake, you can always replace the sugar substitutes with processed sugar and the sugar-free products with regular ones.

I created my recipes knowing they would also be used by hypoglycemics, diabetics, and those concerned about triglycerides. If you choose to use sugar instead, be sure to count the additional calories.

A word of caution when cooking with **sugar substitutes:** Use **saccharin-based** sweeteners when **heating** or **baking**. In recipes that **don't require heat, aspartame** (known as Nutra-Sweet) works well in uncooked dishes but leaves an aftertaste in baked products.

I'm often asked why I use an **8-by-8-inch baking dish** in my recipes. It's for portion control. If the recipe says it serves four, just cut down the center, turn the dish, and cut again. Like magic, there's your serving. Also, if this is the only recipe you are preparing requiring an oven, the square dish fits into an energy-conserving tabletop toaster oven.

To make life even easier, **whenever a recipe calls for ounce measurements** (other than raw meats), I've included the closest cup equivalent. I need to use my scale daily when creating recipes, so I've measured for you at the same time.

Most of the recipes are for **four to six servings**. If you don't have that many to feed, do what I do: freeze individual portions. Then all you have to do is choose something from the freezer and take it to work for lunch or have your evening meals prepared in advance for the week.

In this way, I always have something on hand that is both good to eat and good for me.

Unless a recipe includes hard-boiled eggs, cream cheese, mayonnaise, or a raw vegetable, **the leftovers should freeze well**. (I've marked recipes that freeze well with the symbol of a **snowflake**.) This includes most of the cream pies. Divide any recipe up into individual servings and freeze for your own "TV" dinners.

Unless I specify **"covered" for simmering or baking,** prepare my recipes **uncovered**. Occasionally you will read a recipe that asks you to cover a dish for a time, then to uncover, so read the directions carefully to avoid confusion — and to get the best results.

Low-fat cooking spray is another blessing in a Healthy Exchanges kitchen. It's currently available in three flavors:

- OLIVE-OIL FLAVORED when cooking Mexican, Italian or Greek dishes
- BUTTER FLAVORED when the hint of butter is desired
- REGULAR for everything else

A quick spray of butter-flavored makes air-popped popcorn a low-fat taste treat, or try it as a butter substitute on steaming hot corn on the cob. One light spray of the skillet when browning meat will convince you that you're using "old-fashioned fat," and a quick coating of the casserole dish before you add the ingredients will make serving easier and cleanup quicker.

I use **reduced-sodium canned chicken broth** in place of dry bouillon to lower the sodium content. The intended flavor is still present in the prepared dish. As a reduced-sodium beef broth is not currently available (at least not in DeWitt, Iowa), I use the canned regular beef broth. The sodium content is still lower than regular dry bouillon.

Whenever **cooked rice or pasta** is an ingredient, follow the package directions, but eliminate the salt and/or margarine called for. This helps lower the sodium and fat content. It tastes just fine; trust me on this.

When **chunky salsa** is listed as an ingredient, I leave the degree of "heat" up to your personal taste. In our house, I'm considered a wimp. I go for the "mild" while Cliff prefers "extrahot." How do we compromise? I prepare the recipe with mild salsa because he can always add a spoonful or two of the hotter version to his serving, but I can't enjoy the dish if it's too spicy for me.

Proteins

I use eggs in moderation. I enjoy the real thing on an average of three to four times a week. So, my recipes are calculated on using whole eggs.

However, if you choose to use egg substitute in place of the egg, the finished product will turn out just fine and the fat grams per serving will be even lower than those listed.

If you like the look, taste, and feel of **hard-boiled eggs** in salads, but haven't been using them because of the cholesterol in the yolk, I have a couple of alternatives for you: (1) Pour an 8-ounce carton of egg substitute into a medium skillet sprayed with cooking spray. Cover skillet tightly and cook over low heat until substitute is just set, about ten minutes. Remove from heat and let set, still covered, for ten minutes more. Uncover and cool completely. Chop set mixture. This will make about 1 cup of chopped egg. (2) Even easier is to hard-boil "real eggs," toss the yolk away, and chop the white. Either way, you don't deprive yourself of the pleasure of egg in your salad.

In most recipes calling for **egg substitutes,** you can use two egg whites in place of the equivalent of one egg substitute. Just break the eggs open and toss the yolks away. I can hear some of you already saying, "But that's wasteful!" Well, take a look at the price on the egg substitute package (which usually has the equivalent of four eggs in it), then look at the price of a dozen eggs, from which you'd get the equivalent of six egg substitutes. Now, what's wasteful about that?

Whenever I include **cooked chicken** in a recipe, I use roasted white meat without skin. Whenever I include **roast beef or pork** in a recipe, I

111

use the loin cuts because they are much leaner. However, most of the time, I do my roasting of all these meats at the local deli. I just ask for a chunk of their lean roasted meat, 6 or 8 ounces, and ask them not to slice it. When I get home, I cube or dice the meat and am ready to use it in my recipe. The reason I do this is threefold: (1) I'm getting just the amount I need without left-overs; (2) I don't have the expense of heating the oven; and (3) I'm not throwing away the bone, gristle, and fat I'd be cutting away from the meat. Overall, it is probably cheaper to "roast" it the way I do.

Did you know that you can make an acceptable meat loaf without using egg for the binding? Just replace every egg with ¼ cup of liquid. You could use beef broth, tomato sauce, even applesauce, to name just a few alternatives. For a meat loaf to serve six, I always use 1 pound of extralean ground beef or turkey, 6 tablespoons of dried fine bread crumbs, and ¼ cup of the liquid, plus anything else healthy that strikes my fancy at the time. I mix well and place the mixture in an 8-by-8-inch baking dish or 9-by-5-inch loaf pan sprayed with cooking spray. Bake uncovered at 350 degrees for thirty-five to fifty minutes (depending on the added ingredients). You will never miss the egg.

Any time you are **browning ground meat** for a casserole and want to get rid of almost all of the excess fat, just place the uncooked meat loosely in a plastic colander. Set the colander in a glass pie plate. Place in microwave and cook on HIGH for three to six minutes (depending on the amount being browned), stirring often. Use as you would for any casserole. You can also chop up onions and brown them with the meat if you want.

Milk and Yogurt

Take it from me — nonfat dry milk powder is great! I *do not* use it for drinking, but I *do* use it for cooking. Three good reasons why:

1. It is very **inexpensive**.

2. It **does not sour** because you use it only as needed. Store the box in your refrigerator or freezer and it will keep almost forever.

3. You can easily **add extra calcium** to just about any recipe without added liquid.

I consider nonfat dry milk powder one of Mother Nature's modern-day miracles of convenience. But do purchase a good national name brand (I like Carnation), and keep it fresh by proper storage.

In many of my pies and puddings, I use nonfat dry milk powder and water instead of skim milk. Usually I call for $2/3$ cup nonfat dry milk powder and $1^1/4$ to $1^1/2$ cups water or liquid. This way I can get the nutrients of two cups of milk, but much less liquid, and the end result is much creamier. Also, the recipe sets up quicker, usually in five minutes or less. So if someone knocks at your door unexpectedly at mealtime, you can quickly throw a pie together and enjoy it minutes later.

You can make your own **"sour cream"** by combining ³/₄ cup plain fat-free yogurt with ¹/₃ cup nonfat dry milk powder. The advantages of doing this are fourfold: (1) the dry milk stabilizes the yogurt and keeps the whey from separating; (2) the dry milk helps to cut the tartness of the yogurt; (3) it's still virtually fat free; and (4) the calcium has been increased by 100 percent. Isn't it great how we can make that distant relative of sour cream a first kissin' cousin by adding the nonfat dry milk powder? Or, if you place 1 cup of plain fat-free yogurt in a sieve lined with a coffee filter, and place the sieve over a small bowl and refrigerate for about six hours, you will end up with a very good alternative for sour cream. To **stabilize yogurt** when cooking or baking with it, just add 1 teaspoon cornstarch to every ³/₄ cup yogurt.

If a recipe calls for **evaporated skim milk** and you don't have any in the cupboard, make your own. For every ¹/₂ cup evaporated skim milk needed, combine ¹/₃ cup nonfat dry milk powder and ¹/₂ cup water. Use as you would evaporated skim milk.

You can also make your own **sugar-free and fat-free sweetened condensed milk** at home. Combine 1¹/₃ cups nonfat dry milk powder and

½ cup cold water in a 2-cup glass measure. Cover and microwave on HIGH until mixture is hot but *not* boiling. Stir in ½ cup Sprinkle Sweet or Sugar Twin. Cover and refrigerate at least four hours. This mixture will keep for up to two weeks in the refrigerator. Use in just about any recipe that calls for sweetened condensed milk.

For any recipe that calls for **buttermilk,** you might want to try Jo's Buttermilk: Blend one cup of water and ⅔ cup dry milk powder (the nutrients of two cups of skim milk). It'll be thicker than this mixed-up milk usually is, because it's doubled. Add 1 teaspoon white vinegar and stir, then let it sit for at least ten minutes.

One of my subscribers was looking for a way to further restrict salt intake and needed a substitute for **cream of mushroom soup**. For many of my recipes, I use Healthy Request Cream of Mushroom Soup, as it is a reduced-sodium product. The label suggests two servings per can, but I usually incorporate the soup into a recipe serving at least four. By doing this, I've reduced the sodium in the soup by half again.

But if you must restrict your sodium even more, try making my Healthy Exchanges **Creamy Mushroom Sauce**. Place 1½ cups evaporated skim milk and 3 tablespoons flour in a covered jar. Shake well and pour mixture into a medium saucepan sprayed with butter-flavored cooking spray. Add ½ cup canned sliced mushrooms, rinsed and drained. Cook over medium heat, stirring often, until mixture thickens. Add any seasonings of your choice. You can use this sauce in any recipe that calls for one (10³/₄-ounce) can of cream of mushroom soup.

Why did I choose these proportions and ingredients?

- 1½ cups evaporated skim milk is the amount in one can.
- It's equal to three milk choices or exchanges.
- It's the perfect amount of liquid and flour for a medium cream sauce.
- 3 tablespoons flour is equal to one bread/ starch choice or exchange.
- Any leftovers will reheat beautifully with a flour-based sauce, but not with a cornstarch base.
- The mushrooms are one vegetable choice or exchange.
- This sauce is virtually fat free, sugar free, and sodium free.

Fruits and Vegetables

If you want to enjoy a **"fruit shake"** with some pizazz, just combine soda water and unsweetened fruit juice in a blender. Add crushed ice. Blend on HIGH until thick. Refreshment without guilt.

You'll see that many recipes use ordinary **canned vegetables**. They're much cheaper than reduced-sodium versions, and once you rinse and drain them, the sodium is reduced anyway. I believe in saving money wherever possible so we can afford the best fat-free and sugar-free products as they come onto the market.

All three kinds of **vegetables — fresh, frozen, and canned —** have their place in a healthy diet. My husband, Cliff, hates the taste of frozen or fresh green beans, thinks the texture is all wrong, so I use canned green beans instead. In this case, canned vegetables have their proper place when I'm feeding my husband. If someone in your family has a similar concern, it's important to respond to it so everyone can be happy and enjoy the meal.

When I use **fruits or vegetables** like apples, cucumbers, and zucchini, I wash them really well and **leave the skin on**. It provides added color, fiber, and attractiveness to any dish. And, because I use processed flour in my cooking, I like to increase the fiber in my diet by eating my fruits and vegetables in their closest-to-natural state.

The next time you warm canned vegetables such as carrots or green beans, drain and heat the vegetables in ¼ cup beef or chicken broth. It gives a nice variation to an old standby.

Here's a simple **white sauce** for vegetables and casseroles without using added fat. Place 1½ cups evaporated skim milk and 3 tablespoons flour in a covered jar. Shake well. Pour into medium saucepan sprayed with butter-flavored cooking spray and cook over medium heat until thick, stirring constantly. Add salt and pepper to taste. You can also add ½ cup canned drained mushrooms and/or 3 ounces (¾ cup) shredded reduced-fat cheese. Continue cooking until cheese melts.

Zip up canned or frozen green beans with **chunky salsa**: ½ cup to 2 cups beans. Heat thoroughly. Chunky salsa also makes a wonderful dressing on lettuce salads. It only counts as a vegetable, so enjoy.

For **gravy** with all the "old time" flavor but without the extra fat, try this almost effortless way to prepare it. (It's almost as easy as opening up a store-bought jar.) Pour the juice off your roasted meat, then set the roast aside to "rest" for about 20 minutes. Place the juice in an uncovered cake pan or other large flat pan (we want the large air surface to speed up the cooling process) and put in the freezer until the fat congeals on top and you can skim it off. Or, if you prefer, use a skimming pitcher purchased at your kitchen gadget store. Either way, measure about 1½ cups skimmed broth and pour into a medium saucepan. Cook over medium heat until heated through, about 5 minutes. In a covered jar, combine ½ cup water or cooled potato broth with 3 tablespoons flour. Shake well. Pour flour mixture into warmed juice. Combine well using a wire whisk. Continue cooking until gravy thickens, about 5 minutes. Season with salt and pepper to taste.

Why did I use flour instead of cornstarch? Because any leftovers will reheat nicely with the flour base and would not with a cornstarch base. Also,

3 tablespoons of flour works out to one bread/ starch exchange. This virtually fat-free gravy makes about 2 cups, so you could spoon about $1/2$ cup gravy on your low-fat mashed potatoes and only have to count your gravy as a $1/4$ bread/starch exchange.

Desserts

Thaw lite whipped topping in the refrigerator overnight. Never try to force the thawing by stirring or using a microwave to soften. Stirring it will remove the air from the topping that gives it the lightness and texture we want, and there's not enough fat in it to survive being heated.

How can I frost an entire pie with just $1/2$ cup of whipped topping? First, I don't use an inexpensive brand. I use Cool Whip Lite or La Creme lite. Make sure the topping is fully thawed. Always spread from the center to the sides using a rubber spatula. This way, $1/2$ cup topping will literally cover an entire pie. Remember, the operative word is *frost*, not pile the entire container on top of the pie!

Here's a way to extend the flavor (and oils) of purchased whipped topping. Blend together $3/4$ cup plain nonfat yogurt and $1/3$ cup nonfat dry milk powder. Add sugar substitute to equal 2 tablespoons sugar, 1 cup Cool Whip Lite and 1 teaspoon of the flavoring of your choice (vanilla, coconut, or almond are all good choices). Gently mix and use as you would whipped topping. The texture is almost a cross between marshmallow cream and whipped cream. This is enough to mound high on a pie.

For a different taste when preparing sugar-free instant pudding mixes, use ³/₄ cup plain fat-free yogurt for one of the required cups of milk. Blend as usual. It will be *thicker and creamier.* And, no, it doesn't taste like yogurt. Another variation for the sugar-free instant vanilla pudding is to use 1 cup skim milk and 1 cup crushed pineapple juice. Mix as usual.

For a special treat that tastes anything but "diet," try placing **spreadable fruit** in a container and microwave for about fifteen seconds. Then pour the melted fruit spread over a serving of nonfat ice cream or frozen yogurt. One table-spoon of spreadable fruit is equal to 1 fruit serv-ing. Some combinations to get you started are apricot over chocolate ice cream, strawberry over strawberry ice cream, or any flavor over vanilla. Another way I use spreadable fruit is to make a delicious **topping for a cheesecake or angel food cake**. I take ¹/₂ cup of fruit and ¹/₂ cup Cool Whip Lite and blend the two together with a teaspoon of coconut extract.

The next time you are making treats for the family, try using **unsweetened applesauce** for some or all of the required oil in the recipe. For instance, if the recipe calls for ¹/₂ cup cooking oil, use up to the ¹/₂ cup in applesauce. It works, and most people will not even notice the differ-ence. It's great in purchased cake mixes, but so far I haven't been able to figure out a way to deep-fat fry with it!

Another trick I often use is to include tiny amounts of "real people" food, such as coconut, but extend the flavor by using extracts. Try it — you will be surprised by how little of the real thing you can use and still feel you are not being deprived.

If you are preparing a pie filling that has ample moisture, just line **graham crackers** in the bottom of a 9-by-9-inch cake pan. Pour the filling over the top of the crackers. Cover and refrigerate until the moisture has enough time to soften the crackers. Overnight is best. This eliminates the added **fats and sugars of a piecrust**.

Many of my pie recipes can be frozen (always check for the symbol to be sure), but it's best to cut the leftover pie into individual servings and place them in individual Ziploc bags before you place them in the freezer. That way, when you need one piece, you can pull only one out instead of thawing the entire pie. If you freeze and thaw a pie more than once, you could end up with a substandard result — and a disappointing dessert!

When **stirring fat-free cream cheese to soften it,** use only a sturdy spoon, never an electric mixer. The speed of a mixer can cause the cream cheese to lose its texture and become watery.

Did you know you can make your own **fruit-flavored yogurt?** Mix 1 tablespoon of any flavor of spreadable fruit spread with ¾ cup plain yogurt. It's every bit as tasty and much cheaper. You can also make your own **lemon yogurt** by combining 3 cups plain fat-free yogurt with 1 tub Crystal Light lemonade powder. Mix well, cover, and store in refrigerator. I think you will be pleasantly surprised by the ease, low cost, and flavor of this "made from scratch" calcium-rich treat. P.S.: You can make any flavor you like by using any of the Crystal Light mixes — Cranberry? Iced tea? You decide.

Sugar-free puddings and gelatins are important to many of my recipes, but if you prefer to avoid sugar substitutes, you could still prepare the recipes with regular puddings or gelatins. The calories will be higher, but you would still be cooking in a low-fat way.

When a recipe calls for **chopped nuts** (and you only have whole ones), who wants to dirty the food processor just for a couple of tablespoons? You could try to chop them on your cutting board, but be prepared for bits and pieces to fly all over the kitchen. I use "Grandma's food processor." I use the biggest nuts I can find, put them in a small glass bowl, and chop them into chunks just the right size using a metal biscuit cutter.

If you have a **leftover muffin** and are looking for something a little different for breakfast, you can make **a "breakfast sundae."** Crumble the muffin into a cereal bowl. Sprinkle a serving of fresh fruit over it and top with a couple of tablespoons of nonfat plain yogurt sweetened with sugar substitute and your choice of extract. The thought of it just might make you jump out of bed with a smile on your face. (Speaking of muffins, did you know that if you fill the unused muffin wells with water when baking muffins, you help ensure more even baking and protect the muffin pan at the same time?)

The secret of making **good meringues** without sugar is to use 1 tablespoon of Sprinkle Sweet or Sugar Twin for every egg white and a small amount of extract. Use ½ to 1 teaspoon for the batch. Almond, vanilla, and coconut are all good choices. Use the same amount of cream of tartar you usually do. Bake the meringue in the same old way. Don't think you can't have meringue pies because you can't eat sugar. You can, if you do it my way. (Remember that egg whites whip up best at room temperature.)

Homemade or Store-Bought?

I've been asked which is better for you, homemade from scratch, or purchased foods. My answer is *both!* They each have a place in a healthy lifestyle, and what that place is has everything to do with you.

Take **piecrusts,** for instance. If you love spending your spare time in the kitchen preparing foods, and you're using low-fat, low-sugar, and reasonably low sodium ingredients, go for it! But if, like so many people, your time is limited and you've learned to read labels, you could be better off using purchased foods.

I know that when I prepare a pie (and I experiment with a couple of pies each week, because this is Cliff's favorite dessert), I use a purchased crust. Why? Mainly because I can't make a good-tasting piecrust that is lower in sugar and fat than the brands I use. Also, purchased piecrusts fit my rule of "If it takes longer to fix than to eat, forget it!"

I've checked the nutrient information for the purchased piecrust against recipes for traditional and "diet" piecrusts, using my computer software program. The purchased crust calculated lower in both fat and calories! I have tried some low-fat and low-sugar recipes, but they just didn't spark my taste buds, or were so complicated you needed an engineering degree just to get the crust in the pie plate.

I'm very happy with the purchased piecrusts in my recipes, because the finished product rarely, if ever, has more than 30 percent of total calories coming from fats. I also believe that we have to prepare foods our families and friends will eat with us on a regular basis and not feel deprived, or we've wasted time, energy, and money.

I could use a purchased "lite" **pie filling,** but instead I make my own. Here I can save both fat and sugar, and still make the filling almost as fast as opening a can. The bottom line: Know what you have to spend when it comes to both time and fat/sugar calories, then make the best decision you can for you and your family. And don't go without an occasional piece of pie because you think it isn't *necessary*. A delicious pie prepared in a healthy way is one of the simple pleasures of life. It's a little thing, but it can make all the difference between just getting by with the bare minimum and living a full and healthy lifestyle.

Many people have experimented with my tip about **substituting applesauce and artificial sweetener for butter and sugar,** but what if you aren't satisfied with the result? One woman wrote to me about a recipe for her grandmother's cookies that called for 1 cup of butter and 1½ cups of sugar. Well, any recipe that depends on as much butter and sugar as this one does is generally not a good candidate for "healthy exchanges." The original recipe needed a large quantity of fat to produce the crisp cookie just like the one Grandma made.

Unsweetened applesauce can be used to substitute for vegetable oil with varying degrees of success, but not to replace butter, lard, or margarine. If your recipe calls for ½ cup of oil or less, and it's a quick bread, muffin, or bar cookie, it should work to replace the oil with applesauce. If the recipe calls for more than ½ cup of oil, then experiment with half oil, half applesauce. You've still made the recipe healthier, even if you haven't removed all the oil from it.

Another rule for healthy substitution: Up to ½ cup of sugar or less can be replaced by *an artificial sweetener that can withstand the heat of baking,* like Sugar Twin or Sprinkle Sweet. If it requires more than ½ cup of sugar, cut the amount needed by

75 percent and use ½ cup sugar substitute and sugar for the rest. Other options: Reduce the butter and sugar by 25 percent and see if the finished product still satisfies you in taste and appearance. Or, make the cookies just as Grandma did, realizing they are part of your family's holiday tradition. Enjoy a moderate serving of a couple of cookies once or twice during the season, and just forget about them the rest of the year.

I'm sure you'll add to this list of cooking tips as you begin preparing Healthy Exchanges recipes and discover how easy it can be to adapt your own favorite recipes using these ideas and your own common sense.

A Peek into My Pantry and My Favorite Brands

Everyone asks me what foods I keep on hand and what brands I use. There are lots of good products on the grocery shelves today — many more than we dreamed about even a year or two ago. And I can't wait to see what's out there twelve months from now. The following are my staples and, where appropriate, my favorites *at this time*. I feel these products are healthier, tastier, easy to get — and deliver the most flavor for the least amount of fat, sugar, or calories. If you find others you like as well *or better*, please use them. This is only a guide to make your grocery shopping and cooking easier.

Fat-free plain yogurt (*Yoplait*)

Nonfat dry skim milk powder (*Carnation*)

Evaporated skim milk (*Carnation*)

Skim milk

Fat-free cottage cheese

Fat-free cream cheese (*Philadelphia*)

Fat-free mayonnaise (*Kraft*)

Fat-free salad dressings (*Kraft*)

Fat-free sour cream (*Land O Lakes*)

Reduced-calorie margarine (*Weight Watchers, Smart Beat, or Promise*)

Cooking spray
  Butter flavored (*Weight Watchers*)
  Olive oil flavored and regular (*Pam*)

Vegetable oil (*Puritan Canola Oil*)

Reduced-calorie whipped topping (*Cool Whip Lite or La Creme lite*)

Sugar substitute
  if no heating is involved (*Equal*)
  if heating is required
      white (*Sugar Twin or Sprinkle Sweet*)
      brown (*Brown Sugar Twin*)

Sugar-free gelatin and pudding mixes (*JELL-O*)

Baking mix (*Bisquick Reduced Fat*)

Pancake mix (*Hungry Jack Extra Lights or Aunt Jemima Reduced Calorie*)

Reduced-calorie syrup (*Cary's Sugar Free Maple*)

Parmesan cheese (*Kraft's Fat-Free Topping*)

Reduced-fat cheese (*Kraft, Healthy Favorites, and Weight Watchers*)

Shredded frozen potatoes (*Mr. Dell's*)

Spreadable fruit (*Smucker's, Welch's or Sorrell Ridge*)

Peanut butter (*Peter Pan reduced fat, Jif reduced fat, or Skippy reduced fat*)

Chicken broth (*Campbell's Healthy Request*)

Beef broth (*Swanson*)

Tomato sauce (*Hunt's — Regular and Chunky*)

Canned soups (*Campbell's Healthy Request*)

Tomato juice (*Campbell's Healthy Request*)

Catsup (*Campbell's Healthy Request or Heinz Lite Harvest*)

Purchased piecrust
unbaked (*Pillsbury — from dairy case*)
graham cracker, butter flavored, or chocolate flavored (*Keebler*)

90 percent lean pastrami or corned beef (*Carl Buddig*)

Luncheon meats (*Healthy Choice*)

97 percent fat-free reduced-sodium ham (*Dubuque*)

Lean frankfurters and Polish kielbasa sausage (*Healthy Choice*)

Canned white chicken, packed in water (*Swanson*)

90 percent lean ground turkey

90 percent lean ground beef

Canned tuna, packed in water (*Star Kist*)

Soda crackers (*Nabisco Fat-Free Premium*)

Reduced-calorie bread — 40 calories per slice or less (*Colonial or Wonder Bread*)

Hamburger buns — 80 calories each (*Less*)

Rice — instant, regular, brown, and wild

Instant potato flakes (*Betty Crocker Potato Buds*)

Noodles, spaghetti, and macaroni

Salsa (*Chi-Chi's Mild*)

Pickle relish — dill, sweet, and hot dog

Mustard — Dijon, prepared, and spicy

Unsweetened apple juice

Unsweetened applesauce

Frozen fruit — no sugar added

Fresh fruit

Fresh, frozen, and canned vegetables

Spices

Lemon and lime juice

Instant fruit beverage mixes (*Crystal Light*)

Dry dairy beverage mixes (*Nestlé's Quik, and Swiss Miss*)

"Ice cream" (*Well's Blue Bunny Fat-Free and Sugar-Free Dairy Dessert, Weight Watchers*)

If your grocer does not stock these items, why not ask if they can be ordered on a trial basis? If the store agrees to do so, be sure to tell your friends to stop by, so that sales are good enough to warrant restocking the new products. Competition for shelf space is fierce, so only products that sell well stay around.

Soups

Grande Chili-Cabbage Soup ✳

Wait until you try this wonderful combination of chili and cabbage! You'll never miss the meat in this tummy-warming bowl that's as good for you as it is good tasting.

✌ Serves 4 (2 cups)

3 cups coarsely chopped cabbage
½ cup chopped onion
4 cups reduced-sodium tomato juice
1¾ cups (one 15-ounce can) Hunt's Chunky Tomato Sauce
10 ounces (one 16-ounce can) red kidney beans, rinsed and drained
2 teaspoons chili seasoning mix

In a large saucepan sprayed with olive-flavored cooking spray, combine cabbage, onion, tomato juice, and tomato sauce. Stir in kidney beans and chili seasoning mix. Bring mixture to a boil. Lower heat. Cover and simmer 15 minutes or until vegetables are tender, stirring occasionally.

Each serving equals:
DIABETIC: 4 Vegetable • 1 Meat • 1 Starch
213 Calories • 2 gm Fat • 10 gm Protein • 39 gm Carbohydrate • 1496 mg Sodium • 3 gm Fiber
HE: 5½ Vegetable • 1¼ Protein

Vegetable-Bean Soup

A hearty soup based on pinto and kidney beans? *I saw you!* Don't turn your nose up until you try it. It's rich, satisfying, and full of goodness.

❦ Serves 6 (1⅓ cups)

4 cups (two 16-ounce cans) tomatoes, undrained
2 cups water
½ cup finely chopped celery
½ cup chopped onion
2 cups purchased coleslaw mix
1 tablespoon chili seasoning mix
⅛ teaspoon black pepper
1 teaspoon dried parsley flakes
10 ounces (one 16-ounce can) pinto beans, rinsed
   and drained
10 ounces (one 16-ounce can) red kidney beans,
   rinsed and drained

Place undrained tomatoes in blender and process on HIGH 10 to 15 seconds. Pour blended tomatoes into a large saucepan. Stir in water, celery, onion, coleslaw mix, chili seasoning mix, black pepper, and parsley flakes. Add pinto beans and red kidney beans. Mix well to combine. Bring mixture to a boil. Lower heat. Cover and simmer 30 minutes, stirring occasionally.

HINT:

1½ cups shredded cabbage and ½ cup shredded carrots may be used in place of purchased coleslaw mix.

Each serving equals:

DIABETIC: 2½ Vegetable • 1 Meat • 1 Starch
185 Calories • 1 gm Fat • 10 gm Protein • 34 gm Carbohydrate • 864 mg Sodium • 3 gm Fiber
HE: 2⅓ Vegetable • 1⅔ Protein

Homemade
Cream of Mushroom Soup ✳

You'll have this soup on the table almost as fast as you can open a can from the store! A mushroom lover's dream come true.

✌ Serves 4 (1 cup)

2 cups chopped fresh mushrooms
¹/₂ cup chopped onion
¹/₂ teaspoon dried minced garlic
2 cups (one 16-ounce can) Healthy Request Chicken Broth
1 tablespoon reduced-sodium soy sauce
¹/₄ teaspoon black pepper
1¹/₂ cups (one 12-fluid-ounce can) Carnation Evaporated Skim Milk
6 tablespoons all-purpose flour

In a large saucepan sprayed with butter-flavored cooking spray, sauté mushrooms, onion, and minced garlic until mushrooms start to turn limp, about 5 minutes. Add chicken broth. Mix well to combine. Bring mixture to a boil. Lower heat. Stir in soy sauce and black pepper. In a covered jar, combine evaporated skim milk and flour. Shake well to combine. Stir milk mixture into mushroom mixture. Continue cooking, stirring constantly, until mixture thickens, about 5 minutes.

Each serving equals:

DIABETIC: 1 Skim Milk • ¹/₂ Vegetable •
¹/₂ Starch

157 Calories • 1 gm Fat • 11 gm Protein • 26 gm
Carbohydrate • 462 mg Sodium • 1 gm Fiber

HE: 1¹/₄ Vegetable • ³/₄ Skim Milk • ¹/₂ Bread • 8
Optional Calories

Irish Cream of Potato Soup

My Gaelic ancestors would approve of this un-usual potato soup. I guarantee it will make your eyes smile even if you aren't a bit Irish.

✌ Serves 4 (1¼ cups)

> 2 cups (one 16-ounce can) Healthy Request
>   Chicken Broth
> 1 teaspoon dried minced garlic
> ½ cup sliced green onion with tops
> 1 cup shredded cabbage
> 1½ cups (one 12-fluid-ounce can) Carnation
>   Evaporated Skim Milk
> 1 cup skim milk
> 1⅓ cups (3 ounces) instant potato flakes
> ¼ teaspoon black pepper
> 1 teaspoon dried parsley flakes

In a medium saucepan, combine chicken broth and minced garlic. Stir in onion and cabbage. Cook over medium heat, stirring occasionally, until vegetables are tender, about 10 minutes. Add evaporated skim milk, skim milk, potato flakes, black pepper, and parsley flakes. Mix well to combine. Lower heat. Continue cooking, stir-ring often, until mixture thickens, about 3 to 4 minutes.

Each serving equals:

DIABETIC: 1 Starch • 1 Skim Milk • ¹/₂ Vegetable

201 Calories • 1 gm Fat • 13 gm Protein • 35 gm Carbohydrate • 413 mg Sodium • 1 gm Fiber

HE: 1 Bread • 1 Skim Milk • ³/₄ Vegetable • 8 Optional Calories

Depression Potato Soup

This is an updated version of a soup my grandmother served at her boarding house during the Great Depression. It's as inexpensive, filling, and good now as it was then.

✌ Serves 4 (1½ cups)

> *3 cups (15 ounces) diced raw potatoes*
> *1 cup diced onion*
> *1 cup diced celery*
> *Scant ½ cup (¾ ounce) uncooked fine noodles*
> *2 cups water*
> *1½ cups (one 12-fluid-ounce can) Carnation*
>   *Evaporated Skim Milk*
> *1 teaspoon dried parsley flakes*
> *⅛ teaspoon black pepper*

In a large saucepan, combine potatoes, onion, celery, noodles, and water. Cook over medium heat, stirring occasionally, until vegetables are tender, about 15 minutes. Drain, BUT reserve liquid. Return 1 cup of reserved liquid and drained vegetables back to pan. Stir in evaporated skim milk, parsley flakes, and black pepper. Lower heat. Simmer 10 to 15 minutes, stirring occasionally.

Each serving equals:

DIABETIC: 1 Starch • 1 Skim Milk • ½ Vegetable
145 Calories • 1 gm Fat • 4 gm Protein • 30 gm
Carbohydrate • 103 mg Sodium • 1 gm Fiber
HE: 1 Bread • 1 Vegetable • ¾ Skim Milk

Corn-Veggie Chowder

I created this one day when my son Tommy was home from college. He loves cheese but considers most vegetables worth a barely passing grade. He gave this chowder an A+. (If he were only so generous when it came time to do the dishes . . .)

✌ Serves 6 (1⅓ cups)

2 cups (10 ounces) diced raw potatoes
1 cup diced carrots
1 cup diced celery
½ cup chopped onion
2 cups (one 16-ounce can) Healthy Request Chicken Broth
½ cup (one 2.5-ounce jar) sliced mushrooms, drained
2 cups (one 16-ounce can) cream-style corn
1½ cups (one 12-fluid-ounce can) Carnation Evaporated Skim Milk
¾ cup (3 ounces) shredded Kraft reduced-fat Cheddar cheese
⅛ teaspoon black pepper
2 tablespoons Hormel Bacon Bits

In a medium saucepan, combine potatoes, carrots, celery, onion, and chicken broth. Cook over medium heat 15 minutes or until vegetables are tender. Lower heat. Stir in mushrooms, corn, evaporated skim milk, Cheddar cheese, and black pepper. Continue cooking 5 minutes or until cheese melts, stirring often. Just before serving, stir in bacon bits.

Each serving equals:

DIABETIC: 1½ Starch • ½ Vegetable • ½ Meat • ½ Skim Milk

236 Calories • 4 gm Fat • 14 gm Protein • 36 gm Carbohydrate • 710 mg Sodium • 2 gm Fiber

HE: 1 Bread • 1 Vegetable • ⅔ Protein • ½ Skim Milk • ¼ Slider • 1 Optional Calorie

Chunky Chicken Gumbo

✳

When the weather outside is dreary, or you've been battling the wintry winds on icy roads, a hot bowl of soup just seems to "make it all better." This one is especially thick and soothing.

✌ Serves 4 (1½ cups)

½ cup chopped onion
¼ cup chopped green bell pepper
1 cup sliced celery
½ teaspoon dried minced garlic
1¾ cups (one 15-ounce can) Hunt's Chunky
  Tomato Sauce
2 cups (one 16-ounce can) Healthy Request
  Chicken Broth
1 full cup (6 counces) diced cooked chicken breast
1 cup water
⅔ cup (2 counces) uncooked instant rice
1 cup frozen whole kernel corn
1 cup frozen cut green beans or okra
½ teaspoon Tabasco sauce
1 tablespoon Creole seasoning
⅛ teaspoon black pepper

In a large saucepan sprayed with butter-flavored cooking spray, sauté onion, green pepper, and celery until tender, about 10 minutes. Add minced garlic, tomato sauce, chicken broth, chicken, and water. Mix well to combine. Stir in rice, corn, beans, Tabasco sauce, Creole seasoning, and black pepper. Lower heat. Simmer 25 to 30 minutes, stirring occasionally.

Each serving equals:

DIABETIC: 2½ Vegetable • 1½ Meat • 1 Starch
234 Calories • 2 gm Fat • 20 gm Protein • 34 gm
Carbohydrate • 323 mg Sodium • 3 gm Fiber
HE: 2¼ Vegetable • 1½ Protein • 1 Bread • 8
Optional Calories

Chicken-Noodle Soup

The aroma from this soup is better than all the perfume in Paris. Just ask any man!

✌ Serves 4 (1½ cups)

> 4 cups (two 16-ounce cans) *Healthy Request Chicken Broth*
> ½ cup chopped onion
> 1 cup chopped celery
> 1 cup sliced carrots
> Scant 1 cup (1½ ounces) uncooked noodles
> 1 cup (5 ounces) diced cooked chicken breast
> ⅛ teaspoon black pepper
> 1 teaspoon dried parsley flakes

In a large saucepan, combine chicken broth, onion, celery, and carrots. Bring mixture to a boil. Stir in noodles, chicken, black pepper, and parsley flakes. Lower heat. Cover and simmer about 30 minutes or until vegetables and noodles are tender, stirring occasionally.

Each serving equals:

DIABETIC: 1 Meat • 1 Vegetable • ½ Starch

146 Calories • 2 gm Fat • 16 gm Protein • 16 gm Carbohydrate • 535 mg Sodium • 2 gm Fiber

HE: 1¼ Protein • 1¼ Vegetable • ½ Bread • 16 Optional Calories

Pennsylvania Chicken-Corn Soup ✳

This scrumptious soup hit the spot with the men in my family. Cliff, James, and Tommy all gave it two thumbs — no, make that corn kernels — up!

✌ Serves 4 (1¹/₂ cups)

4 cups (two 16-ounce cans) Healthy Request
  Chicken Broth
1¹/₂ cups (8 ounces) diced cooked chicken breast
1 cup chopped onion
1 cup frozen cut green beans
¹/₄ teaspoon black pepper
¹/₄ teaspoon ground thyme
1 cup frozen whole kernel corn
Scant 1 cup (1¹/₂ ounces) uncooked noodles

In a medium saucepan, combine chicken broth, chicken, onion, green beans, black pepper, and thyme. Cook over medium heat, stirring occasionally, until vegetables are tender, about 15 minutes. Add corn and noodles. Mix well to combine. Lower heat. Cover and simmer 10 minutes or until noodles are tender, stirring occasionally.

Each serving equals:

DIABETIC: 2 Meat • 1¹/₂ Starch • ¹/₂ Vegetable
195 Calories • 3 gm Fat • 19 gm Protein • 23 gm Carbohydrate • 278 mg Sodium • 1gm Fiber
HE: 2 Protein • 1 Bread • ¹/₂ Vegetable • 16 Optional Calories

Garden Pasta Fagioli

My daughter-in-law, Pam, said this is as good as soup gets! The "secret" ingredient is the hot sauce.

✌ Serves 6 (1½ cups)

> 8 ounces ground 90% lean turkey or beef
> ½ cup chopped onion
> 2 cups reduced-sodium tomato juice
> 1¾ cups (one 15-ounce can) Swanson Beef Broth
> 1¾ cups (one 15-ounce can) Hunt's Tomato Sauce
> 1 cup shredded carrots
> 1 cup finely chopped celery
> ¾ cup (2¼ ounces) uncooked tiny shell macaroni
> 10 ounces (one 16-ounce can) navy beans, rinsed
> and drained
> 10 ounces (one 16-ounce can) red kidney beans,
> rinsed and drained
> 1½ teaspoons Italian seasoning
> 2 to 3 drops hot Tabasco sauce

In a large saucepan sprayed with olive-flavored cooking spray, brown meat and onion. Stir in tomato juice, beef broth, tomato sauce, carrots, celery, and macaroni. Bring mixture to a boil. Add navy beans, kidney beans, Italian seasoning, and Tabasco sauce. Mix well to combine. Lower heat. Cover and simmer 15 minutes or until vegetables and pasta are tender, stirring occasionally.

Each serving equals:

DIABETIC: 2 Vegetable • 2 Starch • 1$\frac{1}{2}$ Meat
285 Calories • 5 gm Fat • 18 gm Protein • 42 gm
Carbohydrate • 989 mg Sodium • 4 gm Fiber
HE: 2$\frac{2}{3}$ Vegetable • 2$\frac{2}{3}$ Protein • $\frac{1}{2}$ Bread

Hearty Corn Chili ✳

It's amazing what the addition of corn can do for that old standby, chili. It not only adds crunch, it adds eye appeal too!

✌ Serves 4 (1½ cups)

8 ounces ground 90% lean turkey or beef
½ cup chopped onion
¼ cup chopped green bell pepper
1¾ cups (one 14½-ounce can) stewed tomatoes,
* undrained*
2½ cups reduced-sodium tomato juice
1½ cups frozen whole kernel corn
1 teaspoon chili seasoning mix
¼ teaspoon black pepper
¾ cup (¾ ounce) Corn Chex, slightly crushed

In a large saucepan sprayed with olive-flavored cooking spray, brown meat, onion, and green pepper. Stir in undrained stewed tomatoes, tomato juice, corn, chili seasoning mix, and black pepper. Bring mixture to a boil. Lower heat. Simmer 15 to 20 minutes, stirring occasionally. When serving, evenly sprinkle about 3 tablespoons Corn Chex over top of each soup bowl.

Each serving equals:

DIABETIC: 2½ Vegetable • 1½ Meat • 1 Starch
220 Calories • 5 gm Fat • 14 gm Protein • 30 gm
Carbohydrate • 979 mg Sodium • 2 gm Fiber
HE: 2½ Vegetable • 1½ Protein • 1 Bread

Country-Style Vegetable-Beef Soup ✳

The abundance of carrots is what makes this flavorful soup so special. If you're the kind of person who never gets enough vegetables in your vegetable soup, this might become your new favorite.

Serves 4 (1½ cups)

1 cup water
3½ cups (two 15-ounce cans) Swanson Beef Broth
1½ cups (8 counces) diced cooked lean roast beef
3 cups sliced carrots
1 cup chopped celery
½ cup chopped onion
¼ teaspoon black pepper
¼ teaspoon dried minced garlic
1 teaspoon dried parsley flakes
1¾ cups (3 counces) uncooked wide noodles

In a large saucepan, combine water and beef broth. Stir in beef, carrots, celery, onion, black pepper, minced garlic, and parsley flakes. Bring mixture to a boil. Lower heat. Cover and simmer 20 minutes. Add noodles. Mix well to combine. Continue simmering 15 minutes or until vegetables and noodles are tender, stirring occasionally.

HINTS:
1. This is even better reheated the next day.
2. If you don't have leftover cooked roast beef, try preparing this dish with lean leftover roast pork.

Each serving equals:

DIABETIC: 2 Vegetable • 2 Meat • 1 Starch
238 Calories • 5 gm Fat • 23 gm Protein • 25 gm
Carbohydrate • 566 mg Sodium • 3 gm Fiber
HE: 2¼ Vegetable • 2 Protein • 1 Bread • 9
Optional Calories

Chunky Southwestern Soup

Here are all the flavors of the Southwest stirred up in a robust pot of soup. You can actually taste that desert sunshine — or at least I like to think so.

✌ Serves 4 (1½ cups)

> 8 ounces ground 90% lean turkey or beef
> ½ cup chopped onion
> ½ cup chopped green bell pepper
> 1¾ cups (one 15-ounce can) Swanson Beef Broth
> ¾ cup (1½ ounces) uncooked elbow macaroni
> 2 cups reduced-sodium tomato juice
> 2 cups (one 16-ounce can) tomatoes, undrained and coarsely chopped
> 1 tablespoon chili seasoning mix
> 1 cup frozen whole kernel corn
> ¼ cup (1 ounce) sliced ripe olives

In a large saucepan sprayed with olive-flavored cooking spray, brown meat, onion, and green pepper. Add beef broth, macaroni, tomato juice, undrained tomatoes, and chili seasoning mix. Mix well to combine. Bring mixture to a boil, stirring often. Stir in corn and olives. Lower heat. Cover and simmer 15 minutes or until macaroni is tender, stirring occasionally.

Each serving equals:

DIABETIC: 2 Vegetable • 1½ Meat • 1 Starch • ½ Fat

247 Calories • 7 gm Fat • 16 gm Protein • 30 gm Carbohydrate • 1,083 mg Sodium • 3 gm Fiber

HE: 2½ Vegetable • 1½ Protein • 1 Bread • ¼ Fat • 9 Optional Calories

Calico Bean Soup

This soup is worth its weight in beans! (It's also really high in fiber.) Make a big pot of this and freeze it in individual servings. Then, you can always warm one up in the microwave and savor the flavor all over again.

✌ Serves 8 (1¼ cups)

  1 full cup (6 ounces) diced Dubuque 97% fat-free
    ham or any extra-lean ham
  10 ounces (one 16-ounce can) great northern
    beans, rinsed and drained
  10 ounces (one 16-ounce can) pinto beans, rinsed
    and drained
  10 ounces (one 16-ounce can) red kidney beans,
    rinsed and drained
  10 ounces (one 16-ounce can) lima or butter beans,
    rinsed and drained
  1½ cups shredded carrots
  1 cup chopped celery
  ½ cup chopped onion
  4 cups (two 16-ounce cans) Healthy Request
    Chicken Broth
  ⅛ teaspoon black pepper
  ½ teaspoon dried parsley flakes

In a large saucepan, combine ham, beans, carrots, celery, and onion. Add chicken broth, black pepper, and parsley flakes. Bring mixture to a boil. Lower heat. Cover and simmer 30 minutes or until vegetables are tender, stirring occasionally.

Each serving equals:

DIABETIC: 2 Meat • 2 Starch • ¹/₂ Vegetable
205 Calories • 1 gm Fat • 16 gm Protein • 33 gm
Carbohydrate • 425 mg Sodium • 10 gm Fiber
HE: 2 Protein • 1¹/₂ Bread • ³/₄ Vegetable • 8
Optional Calories

Tomato-Potato-Ham Chowder

This chowder is so thick and creamy, you are going to swear it's loaded with butter and cream. But it's not — and you can prove it by stirring up a pot today!

✌ Serves 4 (1½ cups)

> 1¾ cups (one 14½-ounce can) stewed tomatoes, undrained
> ¼ cup chopped onion
> 2 cups (one chopped onion
> 2 cups (one 16-ounce can) Healthy Request Chicken Broth
> 1½ cups (8 ounces) frozen shredded potatoes
> ½ cup frozen peas
> 1 full cup (6 ounces) Dubuque 97% fat-free ham or any extra-lean ham
> 1½ cups (one 12-fluid-ounce can) Carnation Evaporated Skim Milk
> 3 tablespoons all-purpose flour
> ¾ cup (3 ounces) shredded Kraft reduced-fat Cheddar cheese

In a large saucepan, combine undrained stewed tomatoes, onion, and chicken broth. Bring mixture to a boil. Add shredded potatoes, peas, and ham. Mix well to combine. Lower heat and simmer 10 minutes. In a covered jar, combine evaporated skim milk and flour. Shake well to combine. Add milk mixture to soup mixture. Stir in Cheddar cheese. Continue cooking, stirring constantly, until cheese melts and soup thickens, about 5 minutes.

HINTS:
1. Thaw peas by placing in a colander and rinsing under hot water for one minute.
2. Mr. Dell's frozen shredded potatoes work great.

Each serving equals:

DIABETIC: 2 Meat • 1 Starch • 1 Vegetable • 1 Skim Milk

293 Calories • 5 gm Fat • 25 gm Protein • 37 gm Carbohydrate • 998 mg Sodium • 3 gm Fiber

HE: 2 Protein • 1 Bread • 1 Vegetable • ¾ Skim Milk • 18 Optional Calories

Frankfurter-Cabbage Soup ✳

When I served this to my helpers on a brisk fall day, they all agreed that the aroma was irresistible — and the taste was even better!

✌ Serves 4 (1½ cups)

4 cups reduced-sodium tomato juice
2 cups purchased coleslaw mix
½ cup chopped onion
8 ounces diced Healthy Choice 97% fat-free
    frankfurters
1 teaspoon chili seasoning mix
¼ teaspoon black pepper
⅓ cup (1 ounce) uncooked regular rice
1 teaspoon dried parsley flakes

In a large saucepan, combine tomato juice, coleslaw mix, and onion. Bring mixture to a boil. Stir in frankfurters, chili seasoning mix, black pepper, rice, and parsley flakes. Lower heat. Cover and simmer 20 minutes, stirring occasionally.

HINT:
   1¾ cups shredded cabbage and ¼ cup shredded carrots may be used in place of purchased coleslaw mix.

Each serving equals:

DIABETIC: 3 Vegetable • 1 Meat • ½ Starch

141 Calories • 1 gm Fat • 10 gm Protein • 23 gm Carbohydrate • 1466 mg Sodium • 2 gm Fiber

HE: 3¼ Vegetable • 1⅓ Protein • ¼ Bread

Savory Salads

Tomato Aspic

So pretty for company, and so tasty and easy, your family will thank you if you make this recipe a regular on your table. (If you've never tasted an "aspic" before, please give this one a try . . . even if the combination of lemon gelatin and tomato sauce seems unusual. You may become a real fan!)

✌ Serves 8

1³/₄ cups (one 15-ounce can) Hunt's Tomato Sauce
1 cup water ☆
2 (4-serving) packages JELL-O sugar-free lemon gelatin
1³/₄ cups (one 15-ounce can) Hunt's Chunky Tomato Sauce
¹/₄ cup finely chopped green onion
³/₄ cup finely chopped celery

In a medium saucepan, combine tomato sauce with ¹/₂ cup water. Bring mixture to a boil. Add dry gelatin. Mix well to dissolve gelatin. Remove from heat. Stir in chunky tomato sauce and remaining ¹/₂ cup water. Place pan on a wire rack and allow to cool 15 minutes. Stir in green onion and celery. Mix gently to combine. Pour mixture into ring mold or 8-by-8-inch glass dish. Refrigerate until firm, about 3 hours. Cut into 8 servings.

HINT:

Garnish with fat-free cottage cheese and chives, if desired. If using, count additional exchanges accordingly.

Each serving equals:

DIABETIC: 2 Vegetable

47 Calories • 0 gm Fat • 3 gm Protein • 9 gm Carbohydrate • 713 mg Sodium • 2 gm Fiber

HE: 2 Vegetable • 10 Optional Calories

Honey Dijon Tomato Salad

Everyone will be impressed with your culinary skills when you present this attractive salad. Only you will know that it took just minutes to prepare.

✌ Serves 4

1 cup shredded lettuce
2 cups chopped fresh tomatoes
$\frac{1}{3}$ cup ($1\frac{1}{2}$ ounces) shredded Kraft reduced-fat mozzarella cheese
2 teaspoons dried parsley flakes
$\frac{1}{4}$ cup Kraft Fat Free Honey Dijon Dressing

For each serving, layer $\frac{1}{4}$ cup shredded lettuce on salad plate. Place $\frac{1}{2}$ cup chopped tomatoes over lettuce. Sprinkle about 2 tablespoons mozzarella cheese and $\frac{1}{2}$ teaspoon parsley flakes over top of tomatoes. Drizzle 1 tablespoon dressing over top. Serve at once.

Each serving equals:

DIABETIC: 1 Vegetable • $\frac{1}{2}$ Meat

75 Calories • 3 gm Fat • 4 gm Protein • 8 gm Carbohydrate • 225 mg Sodium • 1 gm Fiber

HE: $1\frac{1}{2}$ Vegetable • $\frac{1}{2}$ Protein • $\frac{1}{4}$ Slider

Super Salad Bowl

This is so filling you could serve it with pride to the hungriest couch potato quarterback you know . . . even during Super Bowl halftime!

✌ Serves 8 (1 cup)

2 cups chopped fresh broccoli
2 cups chopped fresh cauliflower
1 cup sliced carrots
1 cup sliced celery
¹/₂ cup chopped green bell pepper
2 cups cherry tomatoes
1¹/₂ cups sliced fresh mushrooms
1 cup Kraft Fat Free Italian Dressing
¹/₄ cup Hormel Bacon Bits
2 tablespoons grated Kraft fat-free Parmesan cheese

In a large bowl, combine broccoli, cauliflower, carrots, celery, green pepper, cherry tomatoes, and mushrooms. In a small bowl combine Italian dressing, bacon bits, and Parmesan cheese. Add dressing mixture to vegetable mixture. Mix gently to combine. Cover and refrigerate at least 30 minutes. Gently stir again just before serving.

Each serving equals:

Diabetic: 2¹/₂ Vegetable

85 Calories • 1 gm Fat • 4 gm Protein • 15 gm Carbohydrate • 501 mg Sodium • 2 gm Fiber

HE: 2¹/₂ Vegetable • ¹/₄ Slider • 6 Optional Calories

Carrots and More Salad

If you thought carrot salads were b-o-r-i-n-g, munch on this tasty bowl of sunshine and see if you don't declare this salad E-X-C-I-T-I-N-G!

✌ Serves 6 (²/₃ cup)

1 cup shredded carrots
¹/₂ cup chopped celery
1 cup (2 small) unpeeled diced Red Delicious apples
¹/₄ cup raisins
2 tablespoons (¹/₂ ounce) chopped pecans
¹/₃ cup Kraft fat-free mayonnaise
1 teaspoon lemon juice
Sugar substitute to equal 2 teaspoons sugar
¹/₂ teaspoon apple pie spice

In a medium bowl, combine carrots, celery, apples, raisins, and pecans. In a small bowl, combine mayonnaise, lemon juice, sugar substitute, and apple pie spice. Add mayonnaise mixture to carrot mixture. Mix gently to combine. Cover and refrigerate at least 1 hour. Gently stir again just before serving.

Each serving equals:

DIABETIC: 1 Fruit

60 Calories • 0 gm Fat • 1 gm Protein • 14 gm Carbohydrate • 126 mg Sodium • 2 gm Fiber

HE: ²/₃ Fruit • ¹/₂ Vegetable • ¹/₃ Fat • 8 Optional Calories

Peanut Butter–Carrot Salad

Peanut butter dressing for carrots? I had a friend who liked to dip her carrot sticks into a jar of peanut butter. This version is just as good, but with a lot less fat and calories. Give it a taste, and you'll agree that peanut butter and carrots are a natural pairing of flavors — tangy and crunchy.

✌ Serves 4 (½ cup)

> 2 cups shredded carrots
> 6 tablespoons raisins
> 3 tablespoons Peter Pan reduced-fat creamy peanut butter
> ¼ teaspoon dried parsley flakes
> ¼ cup Kraft fat-free mayonnaise
> 2 tablespoons skim milk

In a medium bowl, combine carrots and raisins. In a small bowl, combine peanut butter, parsley flakes, mayonnaise, and skim milk. Add peanut butter mixture to carrot mixture. Mix gently to combine. Refrigerate at least 30 minutes. Gently stir again just before serving.

Each serving equals:

DIABETIC: 1 Meat • 1 Fat • 1 Vegetable • 1 Fruit

148 Calories • 4 gm Fat • 4 gm Protein • 24 gm Carbohydrate • 182 mg Sodium • 2 gm Fiber

HE: 1 Vegetable • ¾ Protein • ¾ Fat • ¾ Fruit • 13 Optional Calories

Fall Apple–Nut Slaw

This is a favorite salad, one I created to savor at a picnic under a tree while the leaves were changing into their spectacular fall colors. Pack up this slaw and take a drive to enjoy the scenery. I bet you'll decide it's so tasty you will want to enjoy it all year long.

✌ Serves 8 (³/₄ cup)

> 3 cups purchased coleslaw mix
> 1 cup shredded red cabbage
> 2 cups (4 small) unpeeled diced Red Delicious apples
> ¹/₂ cup (2 ounces) chopped walnuts
> ³/₄ cup Kraft fat-free mayonnaise
> 1¹/₂ teaspoons lemon juice
> Sugar substitute to equal 3 tablespoons sugar

In a large bowl, combine coleslaw mix, red cabbage, apples, and walnuts. In a small bowl, combine mayonnaise, lemon juice, and sugar substitute. Add mayonnaise mixture to cabbage mixture. Mix well to combine. Cover and refrigerate at least 30 minutes. Gently stir again just before serving.

HINT:
> 2¹/₂ cups shredded cabbage and ¹/₂ cup shredded carrots may be used in place of purchased coleslaw mix.

Each serving equals:

DIABETIC: 1 Vegetable • ½ Fruit • 1 Fat

95 Calories • 4 gm Fat • 1 gm Protein • 14 gm Carbohydrate • 196 mg Sodium • 1 gm Fiber

HE: 1 Vegetable • ½ Fruit • ½ Fat • ¼ Protein • 14 Optional Calories

Italian Broccoli Salad

If your budget doesn't permit a quick trip to Europe for dinner (and whose does?), invite your taste buds to take a Roman holiday without leaving home!

✌ Serves 6 (²/₃ cup)

> *3¹/₂ cups chopped fresh broccoli*
> *¹/₂ cup chopped red onion*
> *³/₄ cup (3 ounces) shredded Kraft reduced-fat mozzarella cheese*
> *2 tablespoons Hormel Bacon Bits*
> *¹/₃ cup Kraft fat-free mayonnaise*
> *¹/₄ cup Kraft Fat Free Italian Dressing*
> *Sugar substitute to equal 1 teaspoon sugar*

In a large bowl, combine broccoli, onion, mozzarella cheese, and bacon bits. In a small bowl, combine mayonnaise, Italian dressing, and sugar substitute. Add mayonnaise mixture to broccoli mixture. Mix gently to combine. Refrigerate at least 30 minutes. Gently stir again just before serving.

Each serving equals:

Diabetic: 2 Vegetable • ¹/₂ Meat

82 Calories • 2 gm Fat • 7 gm Protein • 9 gm Carbohydrate • 392 mg Sodium • 2 gm Fiber

HE: 1¹/₃ Vegetable • ²/₃ Protein • ¹/₄ Slider • 1 Optional Calorie

Mixed Bean Salad

A completely convincing "counterfeit" of the traditional bean salad. I've left in all the taste but stirred out all the excess sugar and fat.

✌ Serves 8 (½ cup)

> 2 cups (one 16-ounce can) cut green beans, rinsed and drained
> 10 ounces (one 16-ounce can) red kidney beans, rinsed and drained
> 10 ounces (one 16-ounce can) garbanzo beans, rinsed and drained
> ½ cup (2 ounces) sliced ripe olives
> ¼ cup chopped fresh parsley
> ½ cup Kraft Fat Free Italian Dressing
> ¼ teaspoon dried minced garlic

In a medium bowl, combine green beans, kidney beans, garbanzo beans, olives, and parsley. Add Italian dressing and minced garlic. Mix gently to combine. Cover and refrigerate at least 2 hours. Gently stir again just before serving.

Each serving equals:

DIABETIC: 1 Starch • 1 Meat • ½ Vegetable

129 Calories • 2 gm Fat • 7 gm Protein • 21 gm Carbohydrate • 276 mg Sodium • 2 gm Fiber

HE: 1¼ Protein • ½ Vegetable • ¼ Fat • 4 Optional Calories

Calico Kraut Salad

Do you love sauerkraut salad but skip it because it's usually made with lots of sugar and oil? Try my version. It's still full of flavor, but the "bad stuff" has disappeared without a trace!

✌ Serves 6 (½ cup)

> 1³/₄ cups (one 14¹/₂-ounce can) Frank's Bavarian-style sauerkraut, drained
> 1 cup frozen whole kernel corn, thawed
> ¹/₄ cup chopped green bell pepper
> ¹/₄ cup canned chopped pimiento
> ¹/₄ cup chopped red onion
> ¹/₄ cup Sugar Twin or Sprinkle Sweet

In a medium bowl, combine sauerkraut, corn, green pepper, pimiento, and red onion. Add Sugar Twin. Mix well to combine. Cover and refrigerate at least 2 hours. Gently stir again just before serving.

HINT:
> If you can't find Bavarian sauerkraut, use regular sauerkraut, ¹/₂ teaspoon caraway seeds, and 1 teaspoon Brown Sugar Twin.

Each serving equals:

DIABETIC: 2 Vegetable

52 Calories • 0 gm Fat • 2 gm Protein • 11 gm Carbohydrate • 527 mg Sodium • 1 gm Fiber

HE: ³/₄ Vegetable • ¹/₃ Bread • 4 Optional Calories

White Bean and Tomato Salad

When I threw this salad together, I didn't know what Cliff would think of the combination. He not only ate it with pleasure, he asked for seconds! That's the kind of applause I like to hear.

✌ Serves 4 (½ cup)

> 10 ounces (one 16-ounce can) navy or great
>   northern beans, rinsed and drained
> 2 tablespoons Hormel Bacon Bits
> ¼ cup chopped green bell pepper
> 2 tablespoons chopped green onion
> ¼ cup (1 ounce) sliced ripe olives
> 1 cup diced fresh tomato
> ½ teaspoon dried minced garlic
> 2 tablespoons fresh minced parsley
> ¼ teaspoon black pepper
> 2 tablespoons Kraft Fat Free Italian Dressing

In a large bowl, combine beans, bacon bits, green pepper, green onion, olives, and tomato. Add minced garlic, parsley, black pepper, and Italian dressing. Mix gently to combine. Cover and refrigerate at least 30 minutes. Gently stir again just before serving.

Each serving equals:

DIABETIC: 1 Meat • 1 Vegetable • 1 Starch

142 Calories • 2 gm Fat • 8 gm Protein • 23 gm Carbohydrate • 189 mg Sodium • 2 gm Fiber

HE: 1¼ Protein • ½ Vegetable • ¼ Fat • 17 Optional Calories

Marinated Mushrooms

If you love mushrooms, then this easy dish will quickly become a mainstay in your recipe collection. I could eat fresh mushrooms almost every day — how about you?

✌ Serves 4

2 cups fresh whole mushrooms
1 cup hot water
¹/₂ cup Kraft Fat Free Italian Dressing

In a medium saucepan, combine mushrooms and water. Bring mixture to a boil. Drain. Place mushrooms in a small bowl. Pour Italian dressing over hot mushrooms. Stir gently to coat. Cover and refrigerate at least 2 hours. Gently stir again just before serving.

Each serving equals:

DIABETIC: 1 Free Food

20 Calories • 0 gm Fat • 1 gm Protein • 4 gm Carbohydrate • 281 mg Sodium • 1 gm Fiber

HE: 1 Vegetable • 8 Optional Calories

Crunchy Pea Salad

I think you will relish this terrific blend of veggies and cashews — and the wonderful colors will make your plate look like a party.

✌ Serves 8 (³/₄ cup)

> *3 cups frozen peas, thawed*
> *1 cup diced celery*
> *1³/₄ cups chopped cauliflower*
> *¹/₄ cup chopped white onion*
> *¹/₂ cup (2 ounces) chopped dry-roasted cashews*
> *2 tablespoons Hormel Bacon Bits*
> *¹/₄ cup Kraft Fat Free Ranch Dressing*
> *¹/₂ cup Kraft fat-free mayonnaise*
> *2 teaspoons dried parsley flakes*
> *Sugar substitute to equal 1 tablespoon sugar*

In a large bowl, combine peas, celery, cauliflower, onion, cashews, and bacon bits. In a small bowl, combine Ranch dressing, mayonnaise, parsley flakes, and sugar substitute. Add dressing mixture to pea mixture. Mix gently to combine. Cover and refrigerate at least 30 minutes. Gently stir again just before serving.

HINT:
  Thaw peas by placing in a colander and rinsing under hot water for one minute.

Each serving equals:

DIABETIC: 1 Starch • 1 Vegetable • ¹/₂ Fat

127 Calories • 4 gm Fat • 5 gm Protein • 18 gm Carbohydrate • 360 mg Sodium • 2 gm Fiber

HE: ³/₄ Bread • ³/₄ Vegetable • ¹/₂ Fat • ¹/₄ Protein • ¹/₄ Slider • 9 Optional Calories

Grandma's Pea Salad

I can't remember a family potluck when my grandmother didn't bring a big dish of her famous pea salad. My version tastes almost exactly the same, and now I bring a big dish of this to our family potlucks. That's how great traditions get started.

✌ Serves 4 (full ½ cup)

2 cups (one 16-ounce can) small peas, rinsed and drained
2 tablespoons chopped white onion
1 tablespoon chopped green bell pepper
½ cup shredded carrots
1 finely diced hard-boiled egg
⅓ cup Kraft fat-free mayonnaise
2 teaspoons prepared mustard
¼ teaspoon black pepper

In a medium bowl, combine peas, onion, green pepper, carrots, and diced egg. Add mayonnaise, mustard, and black pepper. Mix gently to combine. Cover and refrigerate at least 2 hours. Gently stir again just before serving.

Each serving equals:

DIABETIC: 1 Starch

109 Calories • 2 gm Fat • 6 gm Protein • 17 gm Carbohydrate • 404 mg Sodium • 3 gm Fiber

HE: 1 Bread • ⅓ Vegetable • ¼ Protein (limited) • 11 Optional Calories

Beet-Potato Salad

While Cliff and I went on vacation, I tried an unusual salad with beets and potatoes. You know me, I had to "dissect" it while we were eating so I could duplicate the wonderful flavor when we returned home.

✌ Serves 6 ($^2/_3$ cup)

2$^1/_2$ cups (12 ounces) diced cooked potatoes
1 cup (one 8-ounce can) diced beets, rinsed and drained
$^1/_2$ cup frozen peas
$^1/_3$ cup Kraft Fat Free Ranch Dressing
2 tablespoons Kraft fat-free mayonnaise
$^1/_8$ teaspoon black pepper

In a large bowl, combine potatoes, beets, and peas. In a small bowl, combine Ranch dressing, mayonnaise, and black pepper. Pour dressing mixture over vegetables. Mix gently to combine. Refrigerate at least 30 minutes. Gently stir again just before serving.

Each serving equals:

DIABETIC: 1 Starch • 1 Vegetable

87 Calories • 0 gm Fat • 2 gm Protein • 20 gm Carbohydrate • 265 mg Sodium • 1 gm Fiber

HE: $^2/_3$ Bread • $^1/_3$ Vegetable • $^1/_4$ Slider • 5 Optional Calories

Gina's Potato Salad

I created this for my niece Gina's high school graduation party. You might say the salad graduated with honors — just like Gina.

✌ Serves 6 (³/₄ cup)

3 full cups (16 ounces) diced cooked potatoes
³/₄ cup finely chopped celery
¹/₄ cup finely chopped white onion
¹/₃ cup Kraft fat-free mayonnaise
2 teaspoons prepared mustard
1 tablespoon white vinegar
Sugar substitute to equal 1 tablespoon sugar
2 tablespoons sweet pickle relish
¹/₄ teaspoon black pepper

In a medium bowl, combine potatoes, celery, and onion. In a small bowl, combine mayonnaise, mustard, vinegar, sugar substitute, pickle relish, and black pepper. Add mayonnaise mixture to potato mixture. Mix gently to combine. Cover and refrigerate at least 30 minutes. Gently stir again just before serving.

Each serving equals:

DIABETIC: 1 Starch

92 Calories • 0 gm Fat • 2 gm Protein • 21 gm Carbohydrate • 185 mg Sodium • 1 gm Fiber

HE: ²/₃ Bread • ¹/₃ Vegetable • 15 Optional Calories

German Potato Salad

This "new world ingredients" salad still has all the "old world flavor," but not the sugars and fats.

✌ Serves 6 (²/₃ cup)

> 3 full cups (16 ounces) diced cooked potatoes
> ¹/₂ cup finely chopped celery
> 2¹/₂ teaspoons dried parsley flakes ☆
> ¹/₂ cup chopped white onion
> 3 tablespoons Hormel Bacon Bits
> ²/₃ cup water
> 1 tablespoon all-purpose flour
> ¹/₄ cup white vinegar
> 2 tablespoons Sugar Twin or Sprinkle Sweet
> ¹/₄ teaspoon prepared mustard

In a medium bowl, combine potatoes, celery, and 2 teaspoons parsley flakes. Set aside. In a large skillet sprayed with butter-flavored cooking spray, sauté onion until just tender, about 5 minutes. Add bacon bits and continue cooking 1 minute, stirring often. In a covered jar, combine water, flour, vinegar, Sugar Twin, remaining ¹/₂ teaspoon parsley flakes, and mustard. Shake well to combine. Stir flour mixture into onion mixture. Continue cooking, stirring often, until mixture thickens, about 3 minutes. Remove from heat. Pour hot sauce mixture over potatoes. Mix gently to combine. Serve warm or cold.

Each serving equals:

DIABETIC: 1½ Starch

116 Calories • 1 gm Fat • 3 gm Protein • 24 gm Carbohydrate • 270 mg Sodium • 1 gm Fiber

HE: ⅔ Bread • ⅓ Vegetable • ¼ Slider • 2 Optional Calories

Mexican Potato Salad

Olé! is what your taste buds will cheer after just one bite of this easy potato salad! This quick dish is so full of flavor, you may start dancing right in the kitchen.

✌ Serves 2 (³/₄ cup)

1¹/₂ cups (8 ounces) diced cooked potatoes
3 tablespoons (³/₄ ounce) shredded Kraft fat-free
Cheddar cheese
¹/₄ cup chunky salsa
2 tablespoons Kraft Fat Free Ranch Dressing
1 teaspoon dried parsley flakes

In a large bowl, combine potatoes and Cheddar cheese. In a small bowl, combine salsa, Ranch dressing, and parsley flakes. Add dressing mixture to potato mixture. Mix gently to combine. Refrigerate at least 30 minutes. Gently stir again just before serving.

Each serving equals:

DIABETIC: 2 Starch • ¹/₂ Meat

162 Calories • 2 gm Fat • 7 gm Protein • 29 gm Carbohydrate • 360 mg Sodium • 1 gm Fiber

HE: 1 Bread • ¹/₂ Protein • ¹/₄ Vegetable • ¹/₄ Slider

Shrimp-Tomato Salad

All I can say about this glorious salad is that it received rave reviews from my "official taste testers"! They particularly enjoyed the spicy sauce, with its flavorful ingredients.

✌ Serves 4 (³/₄ cup)

>   1¹/₂ cups diced fresh tomatoes
>   1 (4.5-ounce drained weight) can small shrimp, rinsed and drained
>   2 tablespoons chopped fresh parsley
>   ¹/₄ cup Kraft fat-free mayonnaise
>   1 tablespoon chili sauce
>   1 to 3 drops Tabasco sauce
>   ¹/₂ teaspoon lemon pepper
>   1¹/₂ cups finely shredded lettuce

In a medium bowl, combine tomato, shrimp, and parsley. In a small bowl, combine mayonnaise, chili sauce, Tabasco sauce, and lemon pepper. Add mayonnaise mixture to tomato mixture. Mix gently to combine. Refrigerate at least 30 minutes. Just before serving, stir in shredded lettuce.

Each serving equals:

DIABETIC: 1¹/₂ Vegetable • 1 Meat

58 Calories • less than 1 gm Fat • 7 gm Protein • 7 gm Carbohydrate • 257 mg Sodium • 1 gm Fiber

HE: 1¹/₂ Vegetable • ¹/₂ Protein • 15 Optional Calories

Jambalaya Salad

Did you think jambalaya could only be served hot? Well, not anymore — just taste this refreshing salad that serves up a delicious mélange of tastes in every bite.

✌ Serves 6 (1 cup)

1 cup frozen peas, thawed
2 cups cold cooked rice
1 full cup (6 ounces) diced Dubuque 97% fat-free ham or any extra-lean ham
1 (4.5-ounce drained weight) can small shrimp, rinsed and drained
1 teaspoon dried minced garlic
1 cup chopped fresh tomato
1/2 cup chopped green bell pepper
1/4 cup chopped white onion
1/4 cup chopped fresh parsley
2 tablespoons Hormel Bacon Bits
1 teaspoon Cajun seasoning
1/2 cup Kraft fat-free mayonnaise
2 tablespoons chili sauce

In a large bowl, combine peas, rice, ham, shrimp, minced garlic, tomato, green pepper, and onion. Add parsley, bacon bits, Cajun seasoning, mayonnaise, and chili sauce. Mix gently to combine. Cover and refrigerate at least 30 minutes. Gently stir again just before serving.

HINTS:
1. Thaw peas by placing in a colander and rinsing under hot water for 1 minute.
2. 1⅓ cups uncooked rice usually cook to about 2 cups.

Each serving equals:

DIABETIC: 1½ Starch • 1 Meat

166 Calories • 2 gm Fat • 13 gm Protein • 24 gm Carbohydrate • 469 mg Sodium • 2 gm Fiber

HE: 1 Bread • 1 Protein • ⅔ Vegetable • ¼ Slider • 4 Optional Calories

King's Bounty Tuna Salad

Tuna salads have developed a reputation for being dull — maybe because they're such a diet mainstay. But this easy version is so lively, it truly is "fit for a king"!

❧ Serves 4 (½ cup)

> 1½ cups purchased coleslaw mix
> 1 (6-ounce) can white tuna, packed in water, drained and flaked
> ¼ cup finely diced white onion
> 2 tablespoons sweet pickle relish
> ¼ cup chopped green bell pepper
> ¼ cup (1 ounce) pimiento-stuffed green olives, chopped
> ½ cup Kraft fat-free mayonnaise
> ½ teaspoon lemon juice
> ¼ teaspoon lemon pepper
> 6 small fat-free saltine crackers, coarsely crushed
> Lettuce leaves

In a medium bowl, combine coleslaw mix, tuna, onion, pickle relish, green pepper, and olives. Add mayonnaise, lemon juice, and lemon pepper. Mix well to combine. Refrigerate at least 30 minutes. Just before serving, stir in crushed crackers. Serve on lettuce leaves.

HINT:
1¼ cups shredded cabbage and ¼ cup shredded
carrots may be used in place of purchased
coleslaw mix.

Each serving equals:

DIABETIC: 1½ Meat • ½ Starch • 1 Vegetable
126 Calories • 2 gm Fat • 12 gm Protein • 15 gm
Carbohydrate • 662 mg Sodium • 1 gm Fiber
HE: 1 Vegetable • ¾ Protein • ¼ Fat • ¼ Bread
• ¼ Slider • 4 Optional Calories

Tropical Isle Chicken Salad

Serve this at your next luncheon, and see if you're not elected chairperson of the menu committee by a landslide!

✌ Serves 4 (scant ½ cup)

1½ cups (8 ounces) diced cooked chicken breast
1 cup (one 8-ounce can) crushed pineapple, packed in fruit juice, drained
2 tablespoons (½ ounce) chopped slivered almonds
½ cup chopped celery
¼ cup Kraft fat-free mayonnaise
1 teaspoon Brown Sugar Twin

In a medium bowl, combine chicken, pineapple, almonds, and celery. Add mayonnaise and Brown Sugar Twin. Mix well to combine. Refrigerate at least 30 minutes. Gently stir again just before serving.

HINT:
  It's equally good served on lettuce leaves or as a sandwich filling.

Each serving equals:

DIABETIC: 2 Meat • 1 Fruit

167 Calories • 4 gm Fat • 19 gm Protein • 14 gm Carbohydrate • 182 mg Sodium • 1 gm Fiber

HE: 2 Protein • ½ Fruit • ¼ Vegetable • ¼ Fat • 18 Optional Calories

Big Sur Pasta Salad

Can't you hear the waves beating against the coastline as you stir this recipe in your mind? Just wait until you try it . . . it's even better than you imagined!

✌ Serves 6 (1 cup)

> 3 cups cooked elbow macaroni, rinsed and drained
> 3/4 cup (3 ounces) shredded Kraft reduced-fat Cheddar cheese
> 1 scant cup (4 ounces) diced cooked chicken breast
> 1 full cup (6 ounces) diced Dubuque 97% fat-free ham or any extra-lean ham
> 2 teaspoons dried parsley flakes
> 1/3 cup Kraft Fat Free Thousand Island Dressing
> 2 tablespoons Kraft fat-free mayonnaise
> 1 teaspoon lemon juice
> 1/8 teaspoon black pepper

In a large bowl, combine macaroni, Cheddar cheese, chicken, ham, and parsley flakes. In a small bowl, combine Thousand Island dressing, mayonnaise, lemon juice, and black pepper. Add dressing mixture to macaroni mixture. Mix well to combine. Cover and refrigerate at least 30 minutes. Gently stir again just before serving.

Each serving equals:

DIABETIC: 2 Meat • 1½ Starch

208 Calories • 4 gm Fat • 17 gm Protein • 26 gm Carbohydrate • 514 mg Sodium • 1 gm Fiber

HE: 2 Protein • 1 Bread • ¼ Slider • 5 Optional Calories

Italian Spaghetti Salad

This filling salad went over well with my "meat-and-potatoes" guy! Cliff said it almost tasted like pizza — and that's a neat trick for a healthy salad.

✌ Serves 6 (1 cup)

3 cups cold cooked spaghetti, rinsed and drained
1 cup diced unpeeled zucchini
1 cup chopped carrots
¹/₃ cup (1¹/₂ ounces) sliced ripe olives
2 (2.5-ounce) packages Carl Buddig 90% lean pastrami, shredded
2 tablespoons chopped fresh parsley
³/₄ cup Kraft fat-free mayonnaise
¹/₄ cup Kraft Fat Free Italian Dressing
¹/₄ cup (³/₄ ounce) grated Kraft fat-free Parmesan cheese

In a large bowl, combine spaghetti, zucchini, carrots, olives, pastrami, and parsley. In a small bowl, combine mayonnaise, Italian dressing, and Parmesan cheese. Add mayonnaise mixture to spaghetti mixture. Mix gently to combine. Cover and refrigerate at least 30 minutes. Gently stir again just before serving.

HINT:
2¹/₂ cups broken uncooked spaghetti usually cook to about 3 cups.

Each serving equals:

DIABETIC: 1 Starch • 1 Vegetable • 1 Meat

143 Calories • 3 gm Fat • 8 gm Protein • 21 gm Carbohydrate • 495 mg Sodium • 2 gm Fiber

HE: 1 Bread • 1 Protein • $2/3$ Vegetable • $1/4$ Fat • $1/4$ Slider • 3 Optional Calories

Ham and Blue Cheese Pasta Salad

For all you blue cheese lovers — I know you're out there. Even though this doesn't use chunks of real blue cheese, it sure tastes like it!

✌ Serves 6 (²/₃ cup)

1 full cup (6 ounces) diced Dubuque 97% fat-free ham or any extra-lean ham
¹/₄ cup (1 ounce) chopped walnuts
3 cups cooked shell macaroni, rinsed and drained
¹/₂ cup Kraft Fat Free Blue Cheese Dressing
1 teaspoon dried minced parsley flakes
¹/₈ teaspoon black pepper
¹/₄ cup (³/₄ ounce) grated Kraft fat-free Parmesan cheese

In a medium bowl, combine ham, walnuts, and macaroni. Add blue cheese dressing, parsley flakes, and black pepper. Mix well to combine. Refrigerate at least 30 minutes. Just before serving, stir in Parmesan cheese.

HINT:
2¹/₄ cups uncooked macaroni usually cook to about 3 cups.

Each serving equals:

DIABETIC: 1¹/₂ Starch • 1 Meat • ¹/₂ Fat

188 Calories • 4 gm Fat • 10 gm Protein • 28 gm Carbohydrate • 447 mg Sodium • 1 gm Fiber

HE: 1 Protein • 1 Bread • ¹/₃ Fat • ¹/₄ Slider • 1 Optional Calorie

Frankfurter-Corn Salad

As "All-American" as a salad can get, and just right for a summer picnic. This flavorful blend of franks and corn is something special.

✌ Serves 6 (½ cup)

> 8 ounces diced Healthy Choice 97% fat-free frankfurters
> 3 cups frozen whole kernel corn, thawed
> ¾ cup (3 ounces) shredded Kraft fat-free Cheddar cheese
> 2 tablespoons sweet pickle relish
> 1 teaspoon prepared mustard
> ⅓ cup Kraft fat-free mayonnaise
> ¼ teaspoon black pepper

In a large skillet sprayed with butter-flavored cooking spray, sauté frankfurters until browned. Remove from heat. Place skillet on a wire rack and allow to cool 10 minutes. In a medium bowl, combine cooled frankfurters, corn, and Cheddar cheese. Add pickle relish, mustard, mayonnaise, and black pepper. Mix gently to combine. Cover and refrigerate at least 30 minutes. Gently stir again just before serving.

Each serving equals:

DIABETIC: 1 Meat • 1 Starch

127 Calories • 3 gm Fat • 10 gm Protein • 15 gm Carbohydrate • 643 mg Sodium • 1 gm Fiber

HE: 1½ Protein • 1 Bread • 17 Optional Calories

Sweet Salads

Fruit Cocktail Salad

This is so quick and tasty, I'm sure it will become a family standard in your home just as it has in mine.

✌ Serves 6 (²/₃ cup)

1 (4-serving) package JELL-O sugar-free instant banana pudding mix
¹/₃ cup Carnation Nonfat Dry Milk Powder
³/₄ cup Yoplait plain fat-free yogurt
2 cups (one 16-ounce can) fruit cocktail, packed in fruit juice, undrained
¹/₂ cup Cool Whip Lite
1 cup (1 medium) sliced banana

In a large bowl, combine dry pudding mix and dry milk powder. Add yogurt and undrained fruit cocktail. Mix well to combine. Fold in Cool Whip Lite and sliced banana. Refrigerate at least 15 minutes.

Each serving equals:

DIABETIC: 1 Fruit • ¹/₂ Skim Milk
117 Calories • 1 gm Fat • 3 gm Protein • 24 gm Carbohydrate • 265 mg Sodium • 1 gm Fiber
HE: 1 Fruit • ¹/₃ Skim Milk • ¹/₄ Slider • 10 Optional Calories

Pistachio Fruit Salad

Talk about "perfect couples"! The fresh strawberries and pistachio pudding are just made for each other.

✌ Serves 6 (²/₃ cup)

1 (4-serving) package JELL-O sugar-free instant pistachio pudding mix
²/₃ cup Carnation Nonfat Dry Milk Powder
1 cup (one 8-ounce can) crushed pineapple, packed in fruit juice, drained and liquid reserved ☆
Water
¹/₂ cup Cool Whip Lite
1 cup (1 medium) diced banana
2 cups sliced fresh strawberries
¹/₂ cup (1 ounce) miniature marshmallows

In a large bowl, combine dry pudding mix and dry milk powder. Add enough water to reserved pineapple juice to make 1¹/₄ cups liquid. Add liquid to dry pudding mixture. Mix well using a wire whisk. Blend in Cool Whip Lite. Add pineapple, banana, strawberries, and marshmallows. Mix gently to combine. Refrigerate at least 30 minutes. Gently stir again just before serving.

Each serving equals:

DIABETIC: 1 Fruit • ¹/₂ Skim Milk

125 Calories • 1 gm Fat • 3 gm Protein • 26 gm Carbohydrate • 262 mg Sodium • 1 gm Fiber

HE: 1 Fruit • ¹/₃ Skim Milk • ¹/₄ Slider • 15 Optional Calories

Golden Salad

Is it a fruit salad or is it a vegetable salad? Whatever you decide, you're bound to agree that it's truly delicious!

✌ Serves 8

1 cup (one 8-ounce can) crushed pineapple, packed in fruit juice, undrained
¹/₂ cup water
1 (4-serving) package JELL-O sugar-free orange gelatin
1 tablespoon vinegar
1 cup shredded carrots
¹/₄ cup (1 ounce) chopped pecans
1 cup (one 11-ounce can) mandarin oranges, rinsed and drained
¹/₂ cup Kraft fat-free mayonnaise
Sugar substitute to equal 2 tablespoons sugar
1 teaspoon lemon juice

In a medium saucepan, combine undrained pineapple and water. Bring mixture to a boil. Remove from heat. Add dry gelatin and vinegar. Mix well to dissolve gelatin. Refrigerate 5 minutes. Add carrots, pecans, and mandarin oranges. Mix well to combine. Pour mixture into an 8-by-8-inch glass dish. Refrigerate until firm, about 3 hours. In a small bowl, combine mayonnaise, sugar substitute, and lemon juice. Spread mayonnaise mixture evenly over set gelatin. Cut into 8 servings.

Each serving equals:

DIABETIC: 1 Fruit • ½ Fat

78 Calories • 2 gm Fat • 1 gm Protein • 14 gm Carbohydrate • 160 mg Sodium • 1 gm Fiber

HE: ½ Fat • ½ Fruit • ¼ Vegetable • 16 Optional Calories

Green River Salad

Most of the time, I forget I'm more than a couple of years older than my husband, Cliff. But when I started talking about Green River Cokes, he looked at me with a blank stare. I guess he was too young to enjoy this quirky, tangy taste treat from the late fifties.

✌ Serves 8

> 2 (4-serving) packages JELL-O sugar-free lime gelatin
> 1 cup (one 8-ounce can) crushed pineapple, packed in fruit juice, undrained
> 1 cup water
> ¼ cup (1 ounce) chopped pecans
> 1½ cups Diet Coke

In a medium saucepan, combine dry gelatin, undrained pineapple, and water. Cook over medium heat, stirring often, until mixture starts to boil. Remove from heat. Stir in pecans and Diet Coke. Pour mixture into an 8-by-8-inch glass dish. Refrigerate until firm, about 3 hours. Cut into 8 servings.

Each serving equals:

DIABETIC: ½ Fruit • ½ Fat

47 Calories • 2 gm Fat • 1 gm Protein • 6 gm Carbohydrate • 30 mg Sodium • 1 gm Fiber

HE: ½ Fruit • ½ Fat • 10 Optional Calories

Lime Nut Salad

This is such a light and refreshing salad, it's bound to capture rave reviews every time you serve it. What a delectable way to make sure you're getting your calcium, too.

✌ Serves 6

1 cup (one 8-ounce can) crushed pineapple, packed in fruit juice, undrained
1/2 cup boiling water
1 (4-serving) package JELL-O sugar-free lime gelatin
3/4 cup Yoplait plain fat-free yogurt
1/3 cup Carnation Nonfat Dry Milk Powder
Sugar substitute to equal 2 tablespoons sugar
3/4 cup Cool Whip Lite
1 cup fat-free cottage cheese
1/4 cup (1 ounce) chopped walnuts

In a medium saucepan, combine undrained pineapple and water. Bring mixture to a boil. Remove from heat. Add dry gelatin. Mix well to dissolve gelatin. Refrigerate 30 minutes. In a medium bowl, combine yogurt, dry milk powder, and sugar substitute. Add Cool Whip Lite. Mix gently to combine. Fold yogurt mixture into cooled gelatin mixture. Add cottage cheese and walnuts. Mix gently to combine. Pour mixture into an 8-by-8-inch glass dish. Refrigerate until firm, about 3 hours. Cut into 6 servings.

Each serving equals:

DIABETIC: 1 Meat • 1 Fat • 1 Fruit

160 Calories • 4 gm Fat • 15 gm Protein • 16 gm Carbohydrate • 241 mg Sodium • 1 gm Fiber

HE: $^3/_4$ Protein • $^1/_2$ Fat • $^1/_3$ Fruit • $^1/_3$ Skim Milk • $^1/_4$ Slider • 9 Optional Calories

Seventh Heaven Strawberry Salad

Strawberries are, in my opinion, the most wonderful fruit on earth. I hope you enjoy the pleasant combination of this recipe as much as I do. (Don't you wish strawberry season lasted all year long?)

✌ Serves 8

2 (4-serving) packages JELL-O sugar-free
   strawberry gelatin
1½ cups boiling water
1½ cups Diet 7UP
1 cup chopped celery
1 cup (one 8-ounce can) crushed pineapple, packed
   in fruit juice, drained
3 cups sliced fresh strawberries ☆
¼ cup (1 ounce) chopped pecans
¾ cup Cool Whip Lite

In a medium bowl, combine dry gelatin and boiling water. Mix well to dissolve gelatin. Refrigerate 10 minutes. Add Diet 7UP, celery, pineapple, 2½ cups strawberries, and pecans. Mix gently to combine. Pour mixture into an 8-by-8-inch glass dish. Refrigerate until firm, about 3 hours. Spread Cool Whip Lite evenly over set gelatin and sprinkle reserved strawberries over top. Cut into 8 servings.

Each serving equals:

DIABETIC: 1 Fruit • ¹/₂ Fat

99 Calories • 3 gm Fat • 5 gm Protein • 12 gm Carbohydrate • 57 mg Sodium • 1 gm Fiber

HE: ²/₃ Fruit • ¹/₂ Fat • ¹/₄ Vegetable • ¹/₄ Slider • 5 Optional Calories

Sweetheart Salad

Serve this to anyone you want to call you sweetheart, because that's what you will hear after just one palate-pleasing bite. I created this for a Valentine's Day dinner, but love — and sweet treats — are always in season!

❧ Serves 6 (½ cup)

> 1 (4-serving) package JELL-O sugar-free cherry gelatin
> 1 (4-serving) package JELL-O sugar-free vanilla cook & serve pudding mix
> 1¼ cups water
> 2 cups (one 16-ounce can) tart red cherries, packed in water, drained
> 1 cup (one 8-ounce can) crushed pineapple, packed in fruit juice, drained
> 1 cup Cool Whip Lite

In a medium saucepan, combine dry gelatin, dry pudding mix, and water. Stir in cherries. Cook over medium heat, stirring constantly, until mixture thickens and starts to boil. Place pan on a wire rack and allow to cool completely. When cooled, stir in pineapple and Cool Whip Lite. Cover and refrigerate at least 30 minutes. Gently stir again just before serving.

Each serving equals:

DIABETIC: 1 Fruit • ¹/₂ Starch

117 Calories • 1 gm Fat • 6 gm Protein • 21 gm Carbohydrate • 319 mg Sodium • 1 gm Fiber

HE: 1 Fruit • ¹/₂ Slider

Apple-Cheddar Salad

The pleasant combination of apples and Cheddar cheese has been enjoyed by many generations. Here's my updated version for this generation.

❦ Serves 4 (²/₃ cup)

> 1¹/₂ cups (3 small) unpeeled diced Red Delicious
>   apples
> ¹/₂ cup chopped celery
> ¹/₃ cup (1¹/₂ ounces) shredded Kraft reduced-fat
>   Cheddar cheese
> 2 tablespoons (¹/₂ ounce) chopped walnuts
> ¹/₄ cup Kraft fat-free mayonnaise
> 1 teaspoon lemon juice
> Sugar substitute to equal 2 tablespoons sugar

In a medium bowl, combine apples, celery, Cheddar cheese, and walnuts. In a small bowl, combine mayonnaise, lemon juice, and sugar substitute. Add mayonnaise mixture to apple mixture. Mix well to combine. Cover and refrigerate at least 30 minutes. Gently stir again just before serving.

Each serving equals:

Diabetic: 1 Fruit • ¹/₂ Fat

91 Calories • 3 gm Fat • 3 gm Protein • 13 gm Carbohydrate • 223 mg Sodium • 1 gm Fiber

HE: ³/₄ Protein • ³/₄ Fruit • ¹/₄ Fat • ¹/₄ Vegetable • ¹/₄ Slider • 1 Optional Calorie

Banana Split Salad

I think this will become another one on Cliff's "All-Time-Favorites List." How do I know? Simple — he wanted me to make it again as soon as he tasted it. You know it has to be really good to please a TRUCK DRIVIN' MAN.

✌ Serves 8 (³/₄ cup)

1 (4-serving) package JELL-O sugar-free vanilla cook & serve pudding mix
1 (4-serving) package JELL-O sugar-free strawberry gelatin
1 cup (one 8-ounce can) crushed pineapple, packed in fruit juice, drained and liquid reserved ☆
Water
³/₄ cup Yoplait plain fat-free yogurt
¹/₃ cup Carnation Nonfat Dry Milk Powder
Sugar substitute to equal 2 tablespoons sugar
1 teaspoon vanilla extract
1 cup Cool Whip Lite
2 cups (2 medium) sliced bananas
2 cups sliced fresh strawberries
¹/₄ cup (1 ounce) chopped pecans

In a medium saucepan, combine dry pudding mix and dry gelatin. Add enough water to reserved pineapple juice to make 1 cup liquid. Add liquid to dry pudding mixture. Mix well to combine. Cook over medium heat, stirring constantly, until mixture thickens and starts to boil. Remove from heat. Place pan on a wire rack and allow to cool completely. In a large bowl, combine yogurt, dry milk powder, sugar substitute, and vanilla extract. Blend in Cool Whip Lite. Add pineapple, bananas, strawberries, and pecans. Mix gently to combine. Fold in cooled pudding mixture. Refrigerate at least 30 minutes. Gently stir again just before serving.

Each serving equals:

DIABETIC: 1 Fruit • ½ Fat • ½ Starch

143 Calories • 3 gm Fat • 7 gm Protein • 22 gm Carbohydrate • 170 mg Sodium • 1 gm Fiber

HE: 1 Fruit • ½ Fat • ¼ Skim Milk • ¼ Slider • 16 Optional Calories

Apple-Macaroni Salad

You may wonder about this combination — apples in macaroni salad? But let me assure you that this fantastic salad is as tasty as it is unique.

✌ Serves 6 (²/₃ cup)

> *2 cups cooked elbow macaroni, rinsed and drained*
> *4 (³/₄ ounce) slices Kraft reduced-fat Swiss cheese, shredded*
> *1 cup (2 small) unpeeled diced Red Delicious apples*
> *1 cup chopped celery*
> *¹/₂ cup Kraft fat-free mayonnaise*
> *1 teaspoon lemon juice*
> *Sugar substitute to equal 1 tablespoon sugar*
> *1 teaspoon apple pie spice*

In a medium bowl, combine macaroni, Swiss cheese, apples, and celery. In a small bowl, combine mayonnaise, lemon juice, sugar substitute, and apple pie spice. Add mayonnaise mixture to macaroni mixture. Mix well to combine. Cover and refrigerate at least 30 minutes. Gently stir again just before serving.

HINT:
> 1¹/₂ cups uncooked elbow macaroni usually cook about 2 cups.

Each serving equals:

DIABETIC: 1 Starch • ¹/₂ Meat • ¹/₂ Fruit

159 Calories • 4 gm Fat • 5 gm Protein • 26 gm Carbohydrate • 405 mg Sodium • 1 gm Fiber

HE: ²/₃ Bread • ²/₃ Protein • ¹/₃ Fruit • ¹/₃ Vegetable • 12 Optional Calories

June Bride Raspberry Salad

Yes, this refreshing salad is perfect for a bridal shower, but don't forget to serve some to the groom too. If you love raspberries as much as I do, you'll find all kinds of "special occasions" for this special salad.

✌ Serves 8

> 1 (4-serving) package JELL-O sugar-free raspberry gelatin
> ³/₄ cup boiling water
> 1 cup (one 8-ounce can) crushed pineapple, packed in fruit juice, undrained
> ¹/₄ cup cold water
> 3 cups frozen unsweetened red raspberries
> 1 (8-ounce) package Philadelphia Fat Free Cream Cheese
> 1 cup Cool Whip Lite
> 1 teaspoon almond extract
> Sugar substitute to equal 1 tablespoon sugar
> 3 to 4 drops red food coloring

In a medium bowl, combine dry gelatin and boiling water. Mix well to dissolve gelatin. Add undrained pineapple, water, and frozen red raspberries. Mix gently to combine. Pour mixture into an 8-by-8-inch glass dish. Refrigerate until firm, about 3 hours. In a medium bowl, stir cream cheese with a spoon until soft. Stir in Cool Whip Lite, almond extract, and sugar substitute. Add food coloring. Mix gently to combine. Spread topping mixture evenly over set gelatin. Refrigerate at least 30 minutes. Cut into 8 servings.

Each serving equals:

DIABETIC: 1 Fruit • ¹/₂ Meat

87 Calories • 1 gm Fat • 5 gm Protein • 14 gm Carbohydrate • 198 mg Sodium • 2 gm Fiber

HE: ³/₄ Fruit • ¹/₂ Protein • ¹/₄ Slider

Spring Rhubarb Salad

Rhubarb is a mainstay of spring in Iowa. But you can savor this refreshing recipe wherever you live. (If you've never tried rhubarb, let me warn you — this Midwest treat is better than you can imagine!)

✌ Serves 6

> 3 cups finely cut rhubarb
> 2 (4-serving) packages JELL-O sugar-free strawberry gelatin ☆
> 2 cups water ☆
> 1 cup (one 8-ounce can) crushed pineapple, packed in fruit juice, drained
> 1 cup (2 small) unpeeled chopped Red Delicious apples
> ¹/₄ cup (1 ounce) finely chopped pecans

In a medium saucepan, combine rhubarb, 1 package dry gelatin, and 1 cup water. Cook over medium-low heat, stirring often, until rhubarb is soft, about 15 minutes. Remove from heat. Place pan on a wire rack and allow to cool. In a large saucepan, bring remaining 1 cup of water to a boil. Remove pan from heat. Stir in remaining package of dry gelatin. Mix well to dissolve gelatin. Stir in cooled rhubarb mixture, pineapple, apples, and pecans. Pour mixture into an 8-by-8-inch glass dish. Refrigerate until firm, about 3 hours. Cut into 6 servings.

Each serving equals:

DIABETIC: 1 Fruit • 1 Fat

111 Calories • 3 gm Fat • 3 gm Protein • 18 gm Carbohydrate • 75 mg Sodium • 1 gm Fiber

HE: 1 Vegetable • ²/₃ Fruit • ²/₃ Fat • 13 Optional Calories

Modern-Day Pilgrim's Cranberry Salad

I wonder what the first pilgrims would say after trying this tasty salad. I bet it would be "May I have more, please?" (Or maybe, "It was worth the trip!")

❧ Serves 6

> 1 (4-serving) package JELL-O sugar-free raspberry gelatin
> 1 (4-serving) package JELL-O sugar-free vanilla cook & serve pudding mix
> 1 cup water
> 2 cups fresh cranberries
> ³/₄ cup Yoplait plain fat-free yogurt
> ¹/₃ cup Carnation Nonfat Dry Milk Powder
> Sugar substitute to equal 2 tablespoons sugar
> 1 teaspoon vanilla extract
> ¹/₂ cup Cool Whip Lite
> 2 cups (2 medium) diced bananas

In a medium saucepan, combine dry gelatin and dry pudding mix. Stir in water and cranberries. Cook over medium heat, stirring constantly, until mixture comes to a boil and cranberries soften. Remove from heat. Place pan on a wire rack and allow to cool 30 minutes. In a large bowl, combine yogurt and dry milk powder. Stir in sugar substitute and vanilla extract. Fold in Cool Whip Lite. Add cooled cranberry mixture and diced bananas. Mix gently to combine. Evenly spoon mixture into 6 individual serving dishes. Refrigerate at least 30 minutes.

Each serving equals:

DIABETIC: 1 Fruit • ½ Starch

115 Calories • 1 gm Fat • 4 gm Protein • 23 gm Carbohydrate • 175 mg Sodium • 1 gm Fiber

HE: 1 Fruit • ⅓ Skim Milk • ¼ Slider • 15 Optional Calories

Winter Fruit Salad

Every family needs a salad that depends on fruit that's never out of season, don't you agree?

✌ Serves 6 (²/₃ cup)

1 cup (2 small) unpeeled diced Red Delicious apples
1 cup (one 11-ounce can) mandarin oranges, rinsed and drained
³/₄ cup sliced celery
¹/₄ cup Kraft fat-free mayonnaise
2 tablespoons Peter Pan reduced-fat chunky peanut butter
1 teaspoon lemon juice

In a medium bowl, combine apples, oranges, and celery. In a small bowl, combine mayonnaise, peanut butter, and lemon juice. Add mayonnaise mixture to fruit mixture. Mix gently to combine. Refrigerate at least 30 minutes. Gently stir again just before serving.

Each serving equals:

DIABETIC: 1 Fruit • ¹/₂ Fat

99 Calories • 3 gm Fat • 2 gm Protein • 16 gm Carbohydrate • 122 mg Sodium • 1 gm Fiber

HE: ²/₃ Fruit • ¹/₃ Fat • ¹/₃ Protein • ¹/₄ Vegetable • 8 Optional Calories

Vegetables

Escalloped Carrots and Celery ✳

A new way to prepare those old "diet" standbys. You'll be surprised how "fresh" they taste when cooked in a different style.

✌ Serves 6

3 cups diced carrots
2 cups diced celery
2 cups water
1¹/₂ cups (one 12-fluid-ounce can) Carnation Evaporated Skim Milk
3 tablespoons all-purpose flour
1 cup (two 2.5-ounce jars) sliced mushrooms, drained
1 teaspoon dried parsley flakes
¹/₈ teaspoon black pepper
³/₄ cup (3 ounces) shredded Kraft reduced-fat Cheddar cheese
6 tablespoons (1¹/₂ ounces) dried fine bread crumbs

Preheat oven to 375 degrees. Spray an 8-by-8-inch baking dish with butter-flavored cooking spray. In a medium saucepan, combine carrots, celery, and water. Cover and cook over medium heat 20 to 25 minutes or until vegetables are just tender. Drain. In a covered jar, combine evaporated skim milk and flour. Shake well to combine. Pour milk mixture into a medium saucepan sprayed with butter-flavored cooking spray. Cook over medium heat, stirring constantly, until mixture thickens and starts to boil. Add mushrooms, parsley flakes, and black pepper. Mix well to combine. In prepared baking dish, make 2 alternate layers of vegetables, white sauce, Cheddar cheese, and bread crumbs. Cover and bake 30 minutes. Uncover and continue baking additional 15 minutes. Place baking dish on a wire rack and let set 5 minutes. Cut into 6 servings.

Each serving equals:

DIABETIC: 1 Vegetable • ½ Meat • ½ Starch • ½ Skim Milk

164 Calories • 4 gm Fat • 11 gm Protein • 21 gm Carbohydrate • 331 mg Sodium • 2 gm Fiber

HE: 2 Vegetable • ⅔ Protein • ½ Skim Milk • ⅓ Bread

Maple-Coated Carrots

You may never look at carrots in the same way after preparing them in this easy and tasty way that brings out this vegetable's natural sweetness.

✌ Serves 4 ($^1/_2$ cup)

$^1/_4$ cup Cary's Sugar Free Maple Syrup
1 tablespoon chopped walnuts ($^1/_4$ ounce)
2 cups (one 16-ounce can) sliced carrots, rinsed and drained

In a large skillet, combine maple syrup and walnuts. Bring mixture to a boil. Stir in carrots. Lower heat. Simmer 5 minutes or until mixture is heated through, stirring occasionally.

Each serving equals:

DIABETIC: 1 Vegetable

37 Calories • 1 gm Fat • 1 gm Protein • 6 gm Carbohydrate • 51 mg Sodium • 1 gm Fiber

HE: 1 Vegetable • $^1/_4$ Fat • 19 Optional Calories

Country-Style Green Beans ✳

If you want the flavor of southern cooked beans, but not the excess fats and sugar, I think these tasty beans will fill the bill.

✌ Serves 4 (³/₄ cup)

4 cups frozen or fresh cut green beans
1 cup water
¹/₂ cup chopped onion
2 teaspoons Sugar Twin or Sprinkle Sweet
¹/₂ cup (3 ounces) finely chopped Dubuque 97%
    fat-free ham or any extra-lean ham
¹/₄ teaspoon black pepper

In a large saucepan, combine green beans and water. Add onion, Sugar Twin, ham, and black pepper. Mix well to combine. Bring mixture to a boil. Lower heat. Cover and simmer 45 minutes, stirring occasionally.

Each serving equals:

DIABETIC: 2 Vegetable • ¹/₂ Meat

73 Calories • 1 gm Fat • 6 gm Protein • 10 gm Carbohydrate • 188 mg Sodium • 1 gm Fiber

HE: 2¹/₄ Vegetable • ¹/₂ Protein • 1 Optional Calorie

Dijon Green Beans ✳

The addition of the Dijon mustard makes all the difference in this flavorful, creamy dish that couldn't be easier to stir up.

✌ Serves 4

> 3 cups frozen cut green beans
> 2 cups water
> 1½ cups (one 12-fluid-ounce can) Carnation Evaporated Skim Milk
> 3 tablespoons all-purpose flour
> 2 teaspoons Dijon mustard
> ⅛ teaspoon black pepper

In a large saucepan, combine green beans and water. Cook over medium heat 20 to 25 minutes or until beans are just tender. Drain. Return beans to pan. In a covered jar, combine evaporated skim milk and flour. Shake well to combine. Pour milk mixture over hot beans. Continue cooking, stirring often, until mixture thickens. Stir in mustard and black pepper. Continue cooking 2 to 3 minutes, stirring constantly, until mixture is heated through.

Each serving equals:

DIABETIC: 1½ Vegetable • 1 Skim Milk

129 Calories • 1 gm Fat • 9 gm Protein • 21 gm Carbohydrate • 229 mg Sodium • 1 gm Fiber

HE: 1½ Vegetable • ¾ Skim Milk • ¼ Bread

Cliff's Green Beans and More ✳

I wasn't sure what Cliff's reaction to this combination would be, but he agreed it was a tasty way to serve those good old reliable green beans — and wanted to know how soon I was going to fix them like this again. You can use fresh or frozen beans, but Cliff likes canned the best, so that's what I used.

✌ Serves 6 (1 cup)

> 4 cups (two 16-ounce cans) cut green beans, rinsed and drained
> 20 ounces (two 16-ounce cans) great northern beans, rinsed and drained
> 1/2 cup (3 ounces) finely diced Dubuque 97% fat-free ham or any extra-lean ham
> 1/3 cup water
> 1/2 cup chopped onion
> 1/2 cup chunky salsa
> 2 tablespoons Brown Sugar Twin

In a large saucepan, combine green beans, great northern beans, ham, and water. Stir in onion, salsa, and Brown Sugar Twin. Cook over medium heat 5 minutes, stirring often. Lower heat. Cover and simmer 30 minutes, stirring occasionally.

Each serving equals:

DIABETIC: 2 Vegetable • 1 Meat • 1 Starch

160 Calories • 1 gm Fat • 11 gm Protein • 27 gm Carbohydrate • 428 mg Sodium • 3 gm Fiber

HE: 2 Protein • 1²/₃ Vegetable • 2 Optional Calories

Green Beans in Onion Sauce ✳

If you love onions, this creamy dish that blends them with green beans will tickle your taste buds.

✌ Serves 4 (1 cup)

> *¹/₂ cup finely chopped onion*
> *1¹/₂ cups (one 12-fluid-ounce can) Carnation Evaporated Skim Milk*
> *3 tablespoons all-purpose flour*
> *¹/₄ teaspoon lemon pepper*
> *4 cups (two 16-ounce cans) cut green beans, rinsed and drained*

In a large skillet sprayed with butter-flavored cooking spray, sauté onion until tender, about 5 minutes. In a covered jar, combine evaporated skim milk and flour. Shake well to combine. Pour milk mixture into skillet with onion. Add lemon pepper. Mix well to combine. Stir in green beans. Continue cooking, stirring often, until mixture thickens and beans are heated through, about 5 minutes.

Each serving equals:

DIABETIC: 2 Vegetable • 1 Skim Milk

131 Calories • less than 1 gm Fat • 9 gm Protein • 23 gm Carbohydrate • 449 mg Sodium • 2 gm Fiber

HE: 2¹/₄ Vegetable • ³/₄ Skim Milk • ¹/₄ Bread

Broccoli-Walnut Party Casserole

Don't just save this wonderful broccoli dish for a party. You'll turn any weekday meal into a celebration when this is on the menu.

✌ Serves 6

1 (16-ounce) package frozen chopped broccoli
3 tablespoons all-purpose flour
²/₃ cup Carnation Nonfat Dry Milk Powder
2 cups (one 16-ounce can) Healthy Request Chicken Broth ☆
2¹/₂ cups (3³/₄ ounces) Pepperidge Farm dried bread cubes
1 teaspoon sage
1 teaspoon dried parsley flakes
¹/₃ cup (1¹/₂ ounces) chopped walnuts

Preheat oven to 400 degrees. In a large saucepan, cook broccoli in water until just tender, about 10 minutes. Drain well. Place broccoli in an 8-by-8-inch baking dish sprayed with butter-flavored cooking spray. In a covered jar, combine flour, dry milk powder, and 1¹/₄ cups chicken broth. Shake well to combine. Pour mixture into a medium saucepan sprayed with butter-flavored cooking spray. Cook over medium heat, stirring constantly, until mixture thickens and starts to boil. Pour hot sauce over broccoli. In a large bowl, combine bread cubes, sage, parsley flakes, walnuts, and remaining ³/₄ cup chicken broth. Mix well to combine. Sprinkle mixture evenly over top of broccoli mixture. Bake 20 to 25 minutes or until top is crusty. Place baking dish on a wire rack and let set 5 minutes. Divide into 6 servings.

Each serving equals:

DIABETIC: 1½ Vegetable • 1½ Starch • ½ Fat
185 Calories • 5 gm Fat • 9 gm Protein • 26 gm Carbohydrate • 487 mg Sodium • 3 gm Fiber
HE: 1½ Vegetable • 1 Bread • ½ Fat • ⅓ Skim Milk • ¼ Protein • 6 Optional Calories

Frosted Cauliflower-Broccoli Bake

I'm not trying to "hide" the broccoli in this recipe so Cliff will eat it, but this saucy baked vegetable combo is a tasty and attractive way to enjoy your vitamins and minerals.

✌ Serves 4

1 (16-ounce) package frozen cut broccoli and
  cauliflower blend
1 cup water
$^1/_2$ cup Kraft fat-free mayonnaise
2 teaspoons prepared mustard
$^1/_4$ teaspoon lemon pepper
1 teaspoon dried parsley flakes
$^3/_4$ cup (3 ounces) shredded Kraft reduced-fat
  Cheddar cheese

Preheat oven to 375 degrees. Spray an 8-by-8-inch baking dish with butter-flavored cooking spray. In a medium saucepan, cook broccoli and cauliflower in water about 10 minutes or just until vegetables are tender. Drain. In a large bowl, combine mayonnaise, mustard, lemon pepper, and parsley flakes. Add drained vegetables. Mix gently to combine. Pour mixture into prepared baking dish. Sprinkle Cheddar cheese evenly over top. Bake 20 minutes. Place baking dish on a wire rack and let set 5 minutes. Divide into 4 servings.

Each serving equals:

DIABETIC: 2 Vegetable • 1 Meat

107 Calories • 3 gm Fat • 8 gm Protein • 12 gm Carbohydrate • 475 mg Sodium • 2 gm Fiber

HE: 2 Vegetable • 1 Protein • 16 Optional Calories

Creamy Peas and Corn

I just took two of Cliff's favorite vegetables and stirred them up together in a special cream sauce. He said "thank you" even before he tasted them, then said it again after he took a bite.

✌ Serves 4 (¹/₂ cup)

1 cup frozen whole kernel corn
1 cup frozen peas
¹/₂ cup water
¹/₄ cup Land O Lakes no-fat sour cream
¹/₄ teaspoon dried parsley flakes
2 teaspoons dried onion flakes

In a medium saucepan, combine corn, peas, and water. Cook 5 minutes or until vegetables are just tender. Drain. Return vegetables to pan. Stir in sour cream, parsley flakes, and onion flakes. Mix gently to combine. Serve at once.

Each serving equals:

DIABETIC: 1 Starch

80 Calories • 0 gm Fat • 4 gm Protein • 16 gm Carbohydrate • 24 mg Sodium • 3 gm Fiber

HE: 1 Bread • 15 Optional Calories

Corn and Tomato Combo

So easy and so filling. I think this is a perfect choice to serve with meat loaf.

☙ Serves 4 (½ cup)

½ cup chopped onion
1¾ cups (one 15-ounce can) Hunt's Chunky Tomato Sauce
1 cup frozen whole kernel corn
1 teaspoon chili seasoning mix
1 teaspoon Sugar Twin or Sprinkle Sweet

In a large skillet sprayed with butter-flavored cooking spray, sauté onion until tender, about 5 minutes. Add tomato sauce, corn, chili seasoning mix, and Sugar Twin. Mix well to combine. Lower heat. Cover and simmer 10 minutes, stirring occasionally.

HINT:
   Canned whole kernel corn, rinsed and drained, may be used instead of frozen.

Each serving equals:

DIABETIC: 1½ Vegetable • ½ Starch
97 Calories • 2 gm Fat • 3 gm Protein • 17 gm Carbohydrate • 610 mg Sodium • 2 gm Fiber
HE: 2 Vegetable • ½ Bread • 1 Optional Calorie

Tomato-Zucchini Sauté

Even if you are not a big fan of zucchini, I think you will enjoy this combination that always reminds me of veggie pizza crowned with melted cheese!

✌ Serves 4 (¾ cup)

2 cups sliced unpeeled zucchini
½ cup sliced onion
2 tablespoons Kraft Fat Free Italian Dressing
2 cups peeled and coarsely chopped fresh tomatoes
1 tablespoon chopped fresh parsley
¾ cup (3 ounces) shredded Kraft reduced-fat mozzarella cheese

In a large skillet sprayed with butter-flavored cooking spray, sauté zucchini and onion until just tender, about 5 minutes. Stir in Italian dressing. Add tomatoes and parsley. Mix gently to combine. Sprinkle mozzarella cheese evenly over top. Continue cooking until cheese is melted, about 1 to 2 minutes, stirring occasionally.

Each serving equals:

DIABETIC: 2 Vegetable • 1 Meat
91 Calories • 3 gm Fat • 8 gm Protein • 8 gm Carbohydrate • 233 mg Sodium • 2 gm Fiber
HE: 2¼ Vegetable • 1 Protein

Cottage Cheese–Stuffed Tomatoes

Why not try a change of pace from just plain sliced tomatoes? You may discover you like cottage cheese better than you thought you did!

✌ Serves 2

> *2 ripe fresh tomatoes*
> *1 cup fat-free cottage cheese*
> *2 tablespoons chopped green bell pepper*
> *2 tablespoons chopped green onion*
> *¹/₂ teaspoon dried minced garlic*
> *¹/₄ teaspoon black pepper*

Cut tops off tomatoes. Scoop out seeds and pulp. Turn tomatoes upside down and allow to drain on a paper towel for 2 to 3 minutes. In a medium bowl, combine cottage cheese, green pepper, onion, garlic, and black pepper. Split each tomato into 4 wedges, but DO NOT cut all the way to the bottom. Evenly stuff tomatoes with cottage cheese mixture. Refrigerate at least 30 minutes.

Each serving equals:

DIABETIC: 2 Meat • 1 Vegetable

68 Calories • 0 gm Fat • 9 gm Protein • 8 gm Carbohydrate • 223 mg Sodium • 1 gm Fiber

HE: 1¹/₄ Vegetable • 1 Protein

Farmstead Corn Pudding ✳

This tastes just like traditional corn pudding — all I've changed about it is its healthier preparation.

✌ Serves 6

> 2 cups (one 16-ounce can) cream-style corn
> $1/2$ cup chopped onion
> $1/4$ cup chopped green bell pepper
> $2/3$ cup Carnation Nonfat Dry Milk Powder
> $1/2$ cup water
> 6 tablespoons ($1^1/2$ ounces) dried fine bread crumbs
> $3/4$ cup (3 ounces) shredded Kraft reduced-fat
>   Cheddar cheese
> 2 tablespoons Hormel Bacon Bits

Preheat oven to 350 degrees. Spray an 8-by-8-inch baking dish with butter-flavored cooking spray. In a medium bowl, combine corn, onion, and green pepper. Add dry milk powder and water. Mix well to combine. Stir in bread crumbs, Cheddar cheese, and bacon bits. Pour mixture into prepared baking dish. Bake 50 to 55 minutes. Place baking dish on a wire rack and let set 5 minutes. Divide into 6 servings.

Each serving equals:

DIABETIC: 1½ Starch • 1 Meat

182 Calories • 4 gm Fat • 11 gm Protein • 26 gm Carbohydrate • 494 mg Sodium • 1 gm Fiber

HE: 1 Bread • ⅔ Protein • ⅓ Skim Milk • ¼ Vegetable • 10 Optional Calories

Corn and Macaroni Bake ✳

This wonderful way to prepare scalloped corn is a remake I did for a subscriber to my newsletter. She wanted to get rid of the excess sugars and fats in her favorite recipe but still retain the flavor. The original called for ¼ cup of sugar and a whole stick of margarine. Notice that neither is an ingredient in my version. Cliff smacked his lips more than once while testing this for me.

✌ Serves 6

> 1 cup cooked elbow macaroni, rinsed and drained
> 1 cup frozen whole kernel corn
> 1 cup (one 8-ounce can) cream-style corn
> ³/₄ cup (3 ounces) shredded Kraft reduced-fat
>   Cheddar cheese
> 1 teaspoon dried parsley flakes
> ¹/₄ teaspoon black pepper
> 2 tablespoons Kraft Fat Free Catalina Dressing

Preheat oven to 350 degrees. Spray an 8-by-8-inch baking dish with butter-flavored cooking spray. In a medium bowl, combine macaroni, frozen corn, and cream-style corn. Stir in Cheddar cheese, parsley flakes, black pepper, and Catalina dressing. Pour mixture into prepared baking dish. Bake 30 minutes. Place baking dish on a wire rack and let set 5 minutes. Divide into 6 servings.

HINT:

$^2/_3$ cup uncooked macaroni usually cooks to 1 cup.

Each serving equals:

DIABETIC: 1$^1/_2$ Starch • $^1/_2$ Meat

134 Calories • 2 gm Fat • 7 gm Protein • 22 gm Carbohydrate • 283 mg Sodium • 1 gm Fiber

HE: 1 Bread • $^2/_3$ Protein • 6 Optional Calories

Westward Ho Potatoes

I like to imagine this hearty potato dish being served as those wagon trains headed west so many years ago. Of course, making it now is much easier!

✌ Serves 4 (²/₃ cup)

1²/₃ cups water
1¹/₃ cups (3 ounces) instant potato flakes
¹/₃ cup Carnation Nonfat Dry Milk Powder
1 teaspoon dried parsley flakes
¹/₂ cup frozen whole kernel corn
2 tablespoons Kraft Fat Free French Dressing
¹/₃ cup (1¹/₂ ounces) shredded Kraft reduced-fat
*   Cheddar cheese*
¹/₄ teaspoon black pepper

In a large skillet, bring water to a boil. Remove from heat. Stir in potato flakes and dry milk powder. Mix with a fork until fluffy. Add parsley flakes, corn, French dressing, Cheddar cheese, and black pepper. Mix well to combine. Lower heat. Return skillet to heat. Continue cooking, stirring often, until mixture is heated through and cheese is melted.

HINT:
    2 cups cold mashed potatoes may be substituted for water, potato flakes and dry milk powder.

Each serving equals:

DIABETIC: 1½ Starch • ½ Meat

154 Calories • 2 gm Fat • 8 gm Protein • 26 gm Carbohydrate • 199 mg Sodium • 1 gm Fiber

HE: 1¼ Bread • ½ Protein • ¼ Skim Milk • 10 Optional Calories

Main Dishes

Mexican Bean-Noodle Bake ✳

If you think every main dish has to have meat, are you in for a surprise! Just try this recipe. It is full of goodies, including great taste!

✌ Serves 4

> 10 ounces (one 16-ounce can) pinto beans, rinsed and drained
> 1/2 cup frozen whole kernel corn
> 1/2 cup chunky salsa
> 1 cup (one 8-ounce can) Hunt's Tomato Sauce
> 2 teaspoons chili seasoning mix
> 1/8 teaspoon black pepper
> 1 1/2 cups cooked noodles, rinsed and drained
> 3/4 cup (3 ounces) shredded Kraft reduced-fat Cheddar cheese

Preheat oven to 350 degrees. Spray an 8-by-8-inch baking dish with olive-flavored cooking spray. In a large skillet sprayed with olive-flavored cooking spray, combine pinto beans, corn, salsa, tomato sauce, chili seasoning mix, and black pepper. Cook over low heat 10 to 15 minutes, stirring occasionally. Stir in noodles. Pour mixture into prepared baking dish. Sprinkle Cheddar cheese evenly over top. Bake 20 to 25 minutes. Place baking dish on a wire rack and let set 5 minutes. Cut into 4 servings.

HINT:

1¼ cups uncooked noodles usually cook to about 1½ cups.

Each serving equals:

DIABETIC: 2 Meat • 2 Starch • 1 Vegetable
253 Calories • 5 gm Fat • 15 gm Protein • 37 gm Carbohydrate • 768 mg Sodium • 5 gm Fiber
HE: 2¼ Protein • 1¼ Vegetable • 1 Bread

Bean and Cheese Tacos

And you thought kidney beans were dull and boring. Or you thought spicy Mexican food was too fattening to enjoy without guilt. Not my way.

✌ Serves 4

> 6 ounces (one 8-ounce can) red kidney beans, rinsed and drained
> ½ cup chunky salsa ☆
> 1 teaspoon dried minced garlic
> 4 (6-inch) flour tortillas
> 1 (8-ounce) package Philadelphia fat-free Cream Cheese
> ¼ cup (¾ ounce) grated Kraft fat-free Parmesan cheese
> ¹/₂ cup chopped onion
> 2 teaspoons dried parsley flakes

Preheat oven to 350 degrees. In a small bowl, combine kidney beans, 1 tablespoon salsa, and minced garlic. Mash well, using a fork. Place tortillas on ungreased cookie sheet. Spread about 2 tablespoons bean mixture on half of each tortilla, to within ½-inch of edge. In a medium bowl, stir cream cheese with a spoon until soft. Add Parmesan cheese, onion, and parsley flakes. Mix well to combine. Spread cream cheese mixture evenly over other half of tortilla and fold in half. Quickly spray tops with olive-flavored cooking spray. Bake about 10 minutes or until tortilla begins to brown and filling is hot. For each serving, place 1 tortilla on plate and spoon scant 2 tablespoons salsa over top.

Each serving equals:

DIABETIC: 2 Meat • 2 Starch

202 Calories • 2 gm Fat • 16 gm Protein • 30 gm Carbohydrate • 647 mg Sodium • 5 gm Fiber

HE: 2 Protein • 1 Bread • ½ Vegetable

Cheesy Asparagus-Rice Bake ✳

This combo of cheese, asparagus and rice produces an amazingly rich and filling entree — so good, and good for you, too.

✌ Serves 4

> 2 cups chopped fresh asparagus
> 1 cup water
> 2 cups cooked rice
> 1³/₄ cups (one 15-ounce can) Hunt's Chunky
>   Tomato Sauce
> 2 teaspoons chili seasoning mix
> ³/₄ cup (3 ounces) shredded Kraft reduced-fat
>   Cheddar cheese ☆

Preheat oven to 350 degrees. Spray an 8-by-8-inch baking dish with butter-flavored cooking spray. In a medium saucepan, cook asparagus in water until just tender, about 5 minutes. Drain. Return asparagus to saucepan. Add rice, tomato sauce, chili seasoning mix, and ¹/₂ cup Cheddar cheese. Mix gently to combine. Pour mixture into prepared baking dish. Sprinkle remaining ¹/₄ cup Cheddar cheese evenly over the top. Bake 25 to 30 minutes. Place baking dish on a wire rack and let set 5 minutes. Cut into 4 servings.

HINT:
   1¹/₃ cups uncooked rice usually cook to about
      2 cups.

Each serving equals:

DIABETIC: 2 Vegetable • 1 Starch • 1 Meat

194 Calories • 6 gm Fat • 11 gm Protein • 24 gm
Carbohydrate • 772 mg Sodium • 3 gm Fiber

HE: 2³/₄ Vegetable • 1 Bread • 1 Protein

Impossible Zucchini-Tomato Pie

This is a great way to use up your extra end-of-summer zucchini. In fact, you probably will be begging for your neighbors' extra zucchini to make this again and again.

✌ Serves 6

> 2¹/₂ cups chopped unpeeled zucchini
> 1 cup peeled and chopped fresh tomatoes
> ¹/₂ cup chopped onion
> ¹/₄ cup (³/₄ ounce) grated Kraft fat-free Parmesan cheese
> ²/₃ cup Carnation Nonfat Dry Milk Powder
> ³/₄ cup Bisquick Reduced Fat Baking Mix
> 2 eggs or equivalent in egg substitute
> 1 teaspoon Italian seasoning
> 1 cup water

Preheat oven to 375 degrees. Spray deep dish 10-inch pie plate with olive-flavored cooking spray. Layer zucchini, tomatoes, and onion in prepared pie plate. Sprinkle Parmesan cheese over top. In a blender container, combine dry milk powder, baking mix, eggs, Italian seasoning, and water. Cover and process on HIGH 30 seconds. Pour mixture evenly over vegetables and cheese. Bake 35 to 40 minutes or until knife inserted in center comes out clean. Place pie plate on a wire rack and let set 5 minutes. Cut into 6 servings.

Each serving equals:

DIABETIC: 1 Vegetable • 1 Meat • 1 Starch

135 Calories • 3 gm Fat • 8 gm Protein • 19 gm Carbohydrate • 278 mg Sodium • 2 gm Fiber

HE: 1 Vegetable • $2/3$ Protein ($1/3$ limited) • $2/3$ Bread • $1/3$ Skim Milk

Zucchini Spaghetti

Quick, try this before the zucchini takes over the planet!

✌ Serves 4

> *2 cups diced unpeeled zucchini*
> *¹/₂ cup diced onion*
> *1³/₄ cups (one 15-ounce can) Hunt's Chunky Tomato Sauce*
> *¹/₄ teaspoon dried minced garlic*
> *1 teaspoon Italian seasoning*
> *1 teaspoon Sugar Twin or Sprinkle Sweet*
> *2 cups hot cooked spaghetti, rinsed and drained*
> *¹/₄ cup (³/₄ ounce) grated Kraft fat-free Parmesan cheese*

In a large skillet sprayed with olive-flavored cooking spray, sauté zucchini and onion until tender, about 5 minutes. Add tomato sauce, minced garlic, Italian seasoning, and Sugar Twin. Lower heat. Cover and simmer 10 minutes. For each serving, place ¹/₂ cup spaghetti on plate, spoon about ¹/₂ cup sauce over spaghetti, and sprinkle 1 tablespoon Parmesan cheese over top.

HINT:
> 1¹/₂ cups broken uncooked spaghetti usually cook to about 2 cups.

Each serving equals:

DIABETIC: 3 Vegetable • 1 Starch

165 Calories • 1 gm Fat • 8 gm Protein • 31 gm Carbohydrate • 706 mg Sodium • 3 gm Fiber

HE: 3 Vegetable • 1 Bread • 1/4 Protein • 2 Optional Calories

Fillets with Lemon Rice   ✳

Lemon and fish are such a great combination —
each seems to bring out the best in the other. I
also find that rice, so light and yet still filling, is
a naturally good accompaniment.

✌ Serves 4

> 2 tablespoons reduced-calorie margarine
> 1¹/₃ cups (4 ounces) uncooked instant rice
> ¹/₂ cup chopped onion
> ¹/₂ teaspoon lemon pepper
> 1 teaspoon dried parsley flakes
> 2 tablespoons lemon juice
> 1 cup water
> 16 ounces white fish, cut into 4 pieces
> ¹/₂ teaspoon paprika

Melt margarine in a 1-cup glass measure. Set
aside. In an 8-by-8-inch glass baking dish, combine rice, onion, lemon pepper, parsley flakes,
lemon juice, and water. Wash fish pieces in cold
water and pat dry. Arrange fish over top of rice
mixture. Drizzle melted margarine over top of
fish and sprinkle paprika over top. Cover. Microwave on HIGH (100% power) 10 to 12 minutes
or until fish flakes easily. Place baking dish on a
wire rack and let set, covered, 2 to 3 minutes.
For each serving, evenly spoon about ¹/₂ cup rice
on plate and top with 1 piece of fish.

Each serving equals:

DIABETIC: 3 Meat • 1 Starch • $\frac{1}{2}$ Fat

204 Calories • 4 gm Fat • 23 gm Protein • 19 gm Carbohydrate • 180 mg Sodium • 1 gm Fiber

HE: 2 Protein • 1 Bread • $\frac{3}{4}$ Fat • $\frac{1}{4}$ Vegetable

Open-Face Crab Sandwiches

If you want something both elegant and easy for a quick luncheon for friends, then this is the ideal dish for you. You'll feel as if you're dining by the seaside.

✌ Serves 8

¹/₂ cup Kraft fat-free mayonnaise
1 tablespoon Dijon mustard
4 English muffins, split and toasted
1 (8-ounce) can crabmeat or frozen imitation crab, thawed
1 teaspoon Worcestershire sauce
1 teaspoon dried parsley flakes
8 (³/₄ ounce) slices Kraft reduced-fat Swiss cheese

Preheat oven to broil. In a small bowl, combine mayonnaise and mustard. Spread mayonnaise mixture evenly over muffin halves. In a medium bowl, combine crabmeat, Worcestershire sauce, and parsley flakes. Divide crabmeat mixture evenly over muffins. Top each with 1 slice of Swiss cheese. Place muffin halves on a broiler-proof baking sheet. Broil about 3 minutes or until cheese is melted. Serve at once.

Each serving equals:

DIABETIC: 1½ Meat • 1 Starch

178 Calories • 6 gm Fat • 13 gm Protein • 18 gm Carbohydrate • 736 mg Sodium • 1 gm Fiber

HE: 1½ Protein • 1 Bread • 10 Optional Calories

Tuna-Vegetable Fettuccine ✳

Forget that monotonous tuna noodle casserole you've been making since the year one. Try this mouthwatering version instead.

✌ Serves 4 (1 cup)

1 cup frozen cut broccoli
1 cup frozen sliced carrots
1 cup water
1 (10 ³/₄-ounce) can Healthy Request Cream of Mushroom Soup
¹/₄ cup skim milk
¹/₂ cup (1¹/₂ ounces) grated Kraft fat-free Parmesan cheese
1 teaspoon dried parsley flakes
1 (6-ounce) can tuna, packed in water, drained and flaked
2 cups hot cooked fettuccine, rinsed and drained

In a large saucepan, combine broccoli, carrots, and water. Cook over medium heat until vegetables are just tender, about 8 to 10 minutes. Drain. In same saucepan, combine mushroom soup, skim milk, Parmesan cheese, and parsley flakes. Add tuna. Mix well to combine. Stir in drained vegetables and fettuccine. Lower heat. Simmer 5 minutes or until mixture is heated through, stirring occasionally.

HINT:

1½ cups broken uncooked fettuccine usually cook to about 2 cups.

Each serving equals:

DIABETIC: 2 Starch • 1½ Meat • 1 Vegetable
251 Calories • 3 gm Fat • 21 gm Protein • 35 gm Carbohydrate • 623 mg Sodium • 3 gm Fiber
HE: 1¼ Protein • 1 Bread • 1 Vegetable • ½ Slider • 13 Optional Calories

Tuna Florentine

You just may win the "Chef of the Year" award from your family when you serve this one. Let them be the judge. You'll all come out winners!

✌ Serves 4

> 1 tablespoon + 1 teaspoon reduced-calorie margarine
> $^3/_4$ cup thinly sliced onion
> $^1/_2$ teaspoon dried minced garlic
> $1^3/_4$ cups (one $14^1/_2$-ounce can) stewed tomatoes, undrained
> 1 teaspoon Italian seasoning
> 4 cups fresh torn spinach, stems discarded
> 2 cups cooked noodles, rinsed and drained
> 1 (6-ounce) can white tuna, packed in water, drained and flaked
> $^1/_4$ cup ($^3/_4$ ounce) grated Kraft fat-free Parmesan cheese

Place margarine in a large glass bowl. Stir in onion and garlic. Microwave on HIGH (100% power) 1 to 2 minutes. Stir in undrained stewed tomatoes and Italian seasoning. Continue cooking on HIGH 4 to 5 minutes, stirring once. Set aside. Place spinach in an 8-by-8-inch glass baking dish. Cover and cook on HIGH 3 to 4 minutes. Place spinach in sieve. Thoroughly drain and chop well. Return spinach to baking dish. Add cooked noodles and tuna to tomato mixture.

Mix well to combine. Pour tomato mixture evenly over spinach. Sprinkle Parmesan cheese evenly over top. Microwave on HIGH 4 to 5 minutes, turning dish after 2 minutes. Place baking dish on a wire rack and let set 2 to 3 minutes. Cut into 4 servings.

HINT:
  1³/₄ cups uncooked noodles usually cook to about 2 cups.

Each serving equals:

DIABETIC: 2 Meat • 2 Vegetable • 1 Starch • ¹/₂ Fat

263 Calories • 3 gm Fat • 22 gm Protein • 37 gm Carbohydrate • 621 mg Sodium • 8 gm Fiber

HE: 3¹/₄ Vegetable • 1 Protein • 1 Bread • ¹/₂ Fat

Broccoli-Tuna Casserole

"Real" men may tell you they won't eat broccoli or yogurt, but I bet they'll gobble down this appetizing casserole and still manage to flex their muscles.

✌ Serves 6

2 cups cooked elbow macaroni, rinsed and drained
3 cups frozen cut broccoli, thawed
8 ounces (one 9-ounce can) white tuna, packed in
   water, drained and flaked
1 cup (one 8-ounce can) sliced water chestnuts,
   drained
³/₄ cup (3 ounces) shredded Kraft reduced-fat
   Cheddar cheese
1 (10³/₄-ounce) can Healthy Request Cream of
   Mushroom Soup
³/₄ cup Yoplait plain fat-free yogurt
¹/₃ cup Carnation Nonfat Dry Milk Powder
1 teaspoon cornstarch
1 teaspoon Worcestershire Sauce
¹/₂ teaspoon dried minced garlic
¹/₄ cup (³/₄ ounce) grated Kraft fat-free Parmesan
   cheese

Preheat oven to 350 degrees. Spray an 8-by-8-inch baking dish with butter-flavored cooking spray. In a large bowl, combine macaroni, broccoli, tuna, water chestnuts, and Cheddar cheese. In a medium bowl, combine mushroom soup, yogurt, dry milk powder, cornstarch, Worcestershire sauce, and garlic. Add soup mixture to macaroni mixture. Mix well to combine. Pour mixture into prepared baking dish. Sprinkle Parmesan cheese evenly over top. Cover and bake 30 minutes. Uncover and continue baking 10 minutes. Place baking dish on a wire rack and let set 5 minutes. Cut into 6 servings.

HINT:
  1½ cups uncooked elbow macaroni usually cook to about 2 cups.

Each serving equals:

DIABETIC: 2 Meat • 1½ Starch • 1 Vegetable

244 Calories • 4 gm Fat • 22 gm Protein • 30 gm Carbohydrate • 561 mg Sodium • 3 gm Fiber

HE: 1½ Protein • 1 Bread • 1 Vegetable • ⅓ Skim Milk • ¼ Slider • 7 Optional Calories

Tuna Shortcakes ✳

Just by adding shortcakes to that old classic, creamed tuna, I've created a new main dish your family will designate an instant classic.

✌ Serves 4

> 2 teaspoons dried onion flakes
> 3/4 cup Bisquick Reduced Fat Baking Mix
> 2/3 cup Carnation Nonfat Dry Milk Powder ☆
> 1/2 cup water
> 8 ounces (one 9-ounce can) white tuna, packed in water, drained and flaked
> 3/4 cup Yoplait plain fat-free yogurt
> 1 (10 3/4-ounce) can Healthy Request Cream of Mushroom Soup
> 1 teaspoon cornstarch
> 1/2 cup frozen peas
> 2 tablespoons canned chopped pimiento
> 4 (3/4-ounce) slices Kraft reduced-fat American cheese

Preheat oven to 400 degrees. Spray an 8-by-8-inch baking dish with butter-flavored cooking spray. In a medium bowl, combine onion flakes and baking mix. Add 1/3 cup dry milk powder and water. Mix well to combine. Drop mixture by tablespoon into prepared baking dish to form 4 shortcakes. Bake 10 to 12 minutes or until golden brown. Meanwhile, in a large saucepan, combine tuna, yogurt, mushroom soup, remaining 1/3 cup dry milk powder, cornstarch, peas, and pimiento. Cook over medium-low heat, stirring occasionally, until mixture is heated through. For each serving, split a warm shortcake and place on serving plate, arrange cheese slice on bottom half, spoon ¼ cup tuna mixture over cheese, place top half of biscuit over cheese and spoon about ¼ cup tuna mixture over top. Serve at once.

Each serving equals:

DIABETIC: 2 Meat • 2 Starch • ½ Skim Milk
310 Calories • 6 gm Fat • 29 gm Protein • 35 gm Carbohydrate • 822 mg Sodium • 2 gm Fiber
HE: 2 Protein • 1¼ Bread • ¾ Skim Milk • ½ Slider • 4 Optional Calories

French Onion Chicken Bake ✳

One bite of this ultra-easy chicken dish will convince you that healthy food is indeed tasty food. Does it seem too easy to be good? Just smile, and accept all those compliments from your many fans.

✌ Serves 4

> *2 cups thinly sliced onion*
> *¹/₃ cup Kraft Fat Free French Dressing*
> *16 ounces skinned and boned uncooked chicken breasts, cut into 4 pieces*

Preheat oven to 350 degrees. Arrange onion evenly in bottom of an 8-by-8-inch baking dish. Place French dressing in a small bowl. Coat chicken pieces in dressing. Arrange chicken evenly over onion. Drizzle any remaining dressing over chicken. Cover and bake 30 minutes. Uncover and continue baking an additional 10 to 15 minutes. For each serving, place a chicken piece on plate and evenly spoon onion and "sauce" over top.

Each serving equals:

DIABETIC: 3 Meat • 1 Vegetable

176 Calories • 4 gm Fat • 25 gm Protein • 10 gm Carbohydrate • 247 mg Sodium • 1 gm Fiber

HE: 3 Protein • 1 Vegetable • ¼ Slider • 7 Optional Calories

Chicken with French Salsa

Fat Free French Dressing and grilled chicken? Ooh-la-la, you may be pleasantly surprised by the flavor.

✌ Serves 4

½ cup Kraft Fat Free French Dressing ☆
16 ounces skinned and boned uncooked chicken
    breasts, cut into 4 pieces
1 cup chopped onion
½ cup chopped green bell pepper
½ teaspoon prepared mustard
1 tablespoon Brown Sugar Twin
2 tablespoons chopped fresh parsley
2 cups peeled and chopped fresh tomato

Place ¼ cup French dressing in a small, flat dish. Coat chicken pieces in dressing. Place chicken in a large skillet sprayed with butter-flavored cooking spray. Drizzle any remaining dressing from dish over top of chicken pieces. Cook about 5 to 6 minutes on each side or until chicken is tender. Meanwhile, in another large skillet sprayed with butter-flavored cooking spray, sauté onion and green pepper until vegetables are just tender, about 5 minutes. Add remaining ¼ cup French dressing, mustard, Brown Sugar Twin, and parsley. Lower heat and simmer until chicken is browned. Just before serving, add chopped tomatoes to onion mixture. Cook 2 to 3 minutes, stirring occasionally, or until tomatoes are just heated. For each serving, place a chicken piece on plate and spoon a full ½-cup vegetable mixture over top.

Each serving equals:

DIABETIC: 3 Meat • 2 Vegetable • ½ Starch

198 Calories • 2 gm Fat • 28 gm Protein • 17 gm Carbohydrate • 334 mg Sodium • 2 gm Fiber

HE: 3 Protein • 1¾ Vegetable • ½ Slider • 2 Optional Calories

Easy Asparagus Chicken ✳

This unusual combination brings together some flavors most people associate with expensive restaurants, especially my healthy "hollandaise." Now you can enjoy the best things in life while sitting at your own dining table.

✌ Serves 6

> *16 ounces skinned and boned uncooked chicken breasts, cut into $1/2$-inch strips*
> *4 cups fresh asparagus spears or 2 (10-ounce) packages frozen asparagus, thawed*
> *1 (10 $3/4$-ounce) can Healthy Request Cream of Mushroom Soup*
> *$1/2$ cup Kraft fat-free mayonnaise*
> *1 tablespoon lemon juice*
> *1 teaspoon curry powder (optional)*
> *$3/4$ cup (3 ounces) shredded Kraft reduced-fat Cheddar cheese*

Preheat oven to 375 degrees. Spray an 8-by-8-inch baking dish with butter-flavored cooking spray. In a large skillet sprayed with butter-flavored cooking spray, brown chicken about 3 minutes, stirring frequently. Place asparagus in bottom of prepared baking dish. Arrange browned chicken evenly over asparagus. In a medium bowl, combine mushroom soup, mayonnaise, lemon juice, and curry powder. Pour soup mixture into same skillet used to brown chicken.

Cook over low heat 1 minute, stirring until well blended. Evenly spoon soup mixture over chicken and asparagus. Sprinkle Cheddar cheese evenly over top. Cover and bake 30 minutes. Uncover and continue baking 10 minutes. Place baking dish on a wire rack and let set 5 minutes. Cut into 6 servings.

Each serving equals:

DIABETIC: 2½ Meat • 1 Vegetable • ½ Starch
194 Calories • 6 gm Fat • 24 gm Protein • 11 gm Carbohydrate • 512 mg Sodium • 2 gm Fiber
HE: 2⅔ Protein • 1⅓ Vegetable • ½ Slider • 3 Optional Calories

Swiss Baked Chicken ✳

Who said chicken has to be predictable, dull and boring? You may have started to feel that way, particularly if you're eating less red meat and have gotten into a rut. Try this and see if it doesn't wake up your taste buds.

✌ Serves 6

> *16 ounces skinned and boned uncooked chicken breast, cut into 24 pieces*
> *4 (³/₄-ounce) slices Kraft reduced-fat Swiss cheese, shredded*
> *1³/₄ cups (one 15-ounce can) Hunt's Chunky Tomato Sauce*
> *1 teaspoon Italian seasoning*
> *1 tablespoon all-purpose flour*
> *1 tablespoon Sugar Twin or Sprinkle Sweet*
> *¹/₂ cup (one 2.5-ounce jar) sliced mushrooms, drained and finely chopped*

Preheat oven to 350 degrees. Place chicken pieces in an 8-by-8-inch baking dish. Sprinkle Swiss cheese evenly over chicken. In a small bowl, combine tomato sauce, Italian seasoning, flour, Sugar Twin, and chopped mushrooms. Pour sauce mixture evenly over cheese. Cover and bake 30 minutes. Uncover and continue baking 10 to 15 minutes or until chicken is tender. Place baking dish on a wire rack and let set 5 minutes. Divide into 6 servings.

HINT:
  Good served over pasta, potatoes, or rice.

Each serving equals:

DIABETIC: 3 Meat • 1 Vegetable

174 Calories • 6 gm Fat • 22 gm Protein • 8 gm Carbohydrate • 727 mg Sodium • 1 gm Fiber

HE: 2²/₃ Protein • 1¹/₃ Vegetable • 6 Optional Calories

Chicken à la King ✳

Fit for queens as well as kings, this 1950s classic is a traditional dish that deserves to live forever — as long as it's prepared the Healthy Exchanges way!

✌ Serves 4 (¾ cup)

1 (10 ¾-ounce) can Healthy Request Cream of Chicken Soup
1 cup water
⅓ cup Carnation Nonfat Dry Milk Powder
1 cup (5 ounces) diced cooked chicken breast
½ cup (one 2.5-ounce jar) sliced mushrooms, drained
2 tablespoons canned chopped pimiento
⅛ teaspoon black pepper
½ cup frozen peas
1 chopped hard-boiled egg

In an 8-cup glass measuring bowl, combine chicken soup, water, and dry milk powder. Stir in chicken, mushrooms, pimiento, and black pepper. Cover and microwave on HIGH (100% power) 5 minutes. Remove from microwave. Stir in peas and egg. Re-cover and microwave on HIGH 2 minutes. Place bowl on a wire rack and let set 3 minutes. Gently stir.

HINT:
Good served over potatoes, rice, pasta, or toast.

Each serving equals:

DIABETIC: 1½ Meat • 1 Starch

165 Calories • 5 gm Fat • 16 gm Protein • 14 gm Carbohydrate • 444 mg Sodium • 1 gm Fiber

HE: 1½ Protein • ¼ Skim Milk • ¼ Vegetable • ¼ Bread • ½ Slider • 5 Optional Calories

Pecan Chicken

※

The perfect choice for a dinner "getaway," even if the only "getaway" you manage is a dinner just for two at your own kitchen table.

✌ Serves 2

¹/₂ cup chopped celery
2 cups skim milk
3 tablespoons all-purpose flour
¹/₈ teaspoon poultry seasoning
1 teaspoon lemon juice
1 cup (5 ounces) diced cooked chicken breast
2 tablespoons canned chopped pimiento
¹/₂ cup frozen peas
2 tablespoons (¹/₂ ounce) chopped pecans

In a medium skillet sprayed with butter-flavored cooking spray, sauté celery until tender, about 5 minutes. In a covered jar, combine skim milk, flour, and poultry seasoning. Shake well to combine. Add milk mixture to celery. Continue cooking, stirring constantly, until mixture thickens. Stir in lemon juice, chicken, pimento, peas, and pecans. Continue cooking until mixture is heated through, about 5 minutes.

HINT:
Good served over toast, potatoes, pasta, or pancakes.

Each serving equals:

DIABETIC: 2 Meat • 1 Starch • 1 Skim Milk • 1 Fat

315 Calories • 7 gm Fat • 34 gm Protein • 29 gm Carbohydrate • 208 mg Sodium • 3 gm Fiber

HE: 2½ Protein • 1 Bread • 1 Skim Milk • 1 Fat • ½ Vegetable

Chicken Salad Burritos

Ordinary chicken salad sandwiches will never seem the same after you feast on this easy burrito.

✌ Serves 4

1 cup (5 ounces) diced cooked chicken breast
1 cup diced unpeeled cucumber
³/₄ cup (3 ounces) shredded Kraft reduced-fat Cheddar cheese
¹/₄ cup Kraft Fat Free Ranch Dressing
2 tablespoons Kraft fat-free mayonnaise
1 teaspoon taco seasoning mix
4 (6-inch) flour tortillas
¹/₂ cup finely shredded lettuce

In a medium bowl, combine chicken, cucumber, and Cheddar cheese. In a small bowl, combine Ranch dressing, mayonnaise, and taco seasoning mix. Add dressing mixture to chicken mixture. Toss gently to combine. Spoon ¹/₄ of chicken mixture over each tortilla. Top each with 2 tablespoons shredded lettuce. Roll tortillas to cover filling. Serve at once or cover and refrigerate until ready to serve.

Each serving equals:

DIABETIC: 2 Meat • 1 Starch • 1 Vegetable
237 Calories • 7 gm Fat • 20 gm Protein • 23 gm Carbohydrate • 531 mg Sodium • 1 gm Fiber
HE: 2¹/₄ Protein • 1 Bread • ¹/₂ Vegetable • ¹/₄ Slider • 10 Optional Calories

Chicken Casserole with Potato-Cheese Topping ✳

If you want to impress anyone for any reason, serve this show-stopping dish. Then wait for them to yell encore!

✌ Serves 6

1/2 cup diced onion
1 cup chopped celery
1 cup chopped carrots
2 cups (one 16-ounce can) Healthy Request Chicken Broth
1 1/2 cups (8 ounces) diced cooked chicken breast
1/2 cup frozen peas
1/2 cup (one 2.5-ounce jar) sliced mushrooms, drained
1/4 teaspoon black pepper
1 1/2 cups (one 12-fluid-ounce can) Carnation Evaporated Skim Milk
3 tablespoons all-purpose flour
3 cups (10 ounces) frozen shredded potatoes, thawed
3/4 cup (3 ounces) shredded Kraft reduced-fat Cheddar cheese
2 teaspoons dried parsley flakes

Preheat oven to 375 degrees. Spray an 8-by-8-inch baking dish with butter-flavored cooking spray. In a medium saucepan, cook onion, celery, and carrots in chicken broth until vegetables are tender, about 15 to 20 minutes. Add chicken, peas, mushrooms, and black pepper. Mix well to combine. In a covered jar, combine evaporated skim milk and flour. Shake well to combine. Add milk mixture to chicken mixture. Continue cooking, stirring often, until mixture thickens. Pour chicken mixture into prepared baking dish and set aside. Place potatoes in a large bowl. Add Cheddar cheese and parsley flakes. Mix well to combine. Sprinkle potato mixture evenly over chicken mixture. Cover and bake 30 minutes. Uncover and continue baking 15 minutes. Place baking dish on a wire rack and let set 5 minutes. Cut into 6 servings.

Each serving equals:

DIABETIC: 2 Meat • 1 Starch • ½ Vegetable • ½ Skim Milk

232 Calories • 4 gm Fat • 24 gm Protein • 25 gm Carbohydrate • 458 mg Sodium • 3 gm Fiber

HE: 2 Protein • 1 Vegetable • ⅔ Bread • ½ Skim Milk • 11 Optional Calories

Salsa Chicken–Topped Potato ✳

Just because you may be cooking for only one or two doesn't mean you can't enjoy a festive way to serve baked potatoes. This one makes any lunch or dinner feel special, and the microwave makes it easy to have great baked potatoes — FAST!

Serves 2

2 (5-ounce) baking potatoes
1 cup (5 ounces) finely diced cooked chicken breast
1/2 cup chunky salsa
1 cup (one 8-ounce can) Hunt's Tomato Sauce
1 tablespoon Brown Sugar Twin
2 tablespoons Land O Lakes no-fat sour cream
2 tablespoons chopped fresh parsley

Scrub and prick potatoes with a fork. Place potatoes on microwavable baking sheet. Microwave on HIGH (100% power) 8 to 10 minutes or until potatoes are almost tender, turning after 4 minutes. Let stand to finish cooking while preparing topping. In a 4-cup glass measure, combine chicken, salsa, tomato sauce, and Brown Sugar Twin. Mix well. Cover and microwave on HIGH 3 minutes. For each serving, place 1 potato on plate, slit potato, and spoon about 1 cup sauce over top and garnish with 1 tablespoon sour cream and 1 tablespoon parsley.

Each serving equals:

DIABETIC: 2¹/₂ Meat • 2¹/₂ Vegetable • 1 Starch
247 Calories • 3 gm Fat • 26 gm Protein • 29 gm
Carbohydrate • 1,056 mg Sodium • 4 gm Fiber
HE: 2¹/₂ Protein • 1 Bread • 2¹/₂ Vegetable • 17
Optional Calories

Turkey in the Straw ✳

Every day will seem like the day after Thanksgiving when you serve this wonderful turkey dish.

✌ Serves 6

3/4 cup Bisquick Reduced Fat Baking Mix
2/3 cup Carnation Nonfat Dry Milk Powder
2 eggs or equivalent in egg substitute
1 teaspoon dried parsley flakes
2 teaspoons poultry seasoning
1 cup water
1 1/2 cups (8 ounces) diced cooked turkey breast
1 cup chopped celery
1/2 cup finely chopped onion

Preheat oven to 375 degrees. Spray a deep-dish 10-inch pie plate with butter-flavored cooking spray. In a large bowl, combine baking mix, dry milk powder, eggs, parsley flakes, poultry seasoning, and water. Mix well using a wire whisk. Stir in turkey, celery, and onion. Pour mixture into prepared pie plate. Bake 35 to 40 minutes or until knife inserted in center comes out clean. Place pie plate on a wire rack and let set 5 minutes. Cut into 6 servings.

Each serving equals:

DIABETIC: 2 Meat • 1 Starch

163 Calories • 3 gm Fat • 18 gm Protein • 16 gm Carbohydrate • 266 mg Sodium • 1 gm Fiber

HE: 1 2/3 Protein • 2/3 Bread • 1/2 Vegetable • 1/3 Skim Milk

Ham Steaks with Cherry Sauce ✳

A truly extraordinary dish, this is actually prepared with very ordinary ingredients — but it doesn't look or taste it!

✌ Serves 6

> 1 (4-serving) package JELL-O sugar-free vanilla cook & serve pudding mix
> 1 (4-serving) package JELL-O sugar-free cherry gelatin
> 2 cups (one 16-ounce can) red tart cherries, packed in water, drained and liquid reserved
> Water
> 1/4 teaspoon apple pie spice
> 6 (3-ounce) slices Dubuque 97% fat-free ham or any extra-lean ham

In an 8-cup glass measuring bowl, combine dry pudding mix and dry gelatin. Add enough water to reserved cherry liquid to make 3/4 cup. Add liquid to pudding mixture. Mix well to combine. Cover and microwave on HIGH (100% power) 2 minutes. Stir in cherries and apple pie spice. Re-cover and continue microwaving on HIGH 2 minutes. Mix well. Cover to keep sauce warm while preparing ham. Place 6 ham steaks in large microwavable dish. Cover with waxed paper. Microwave on HIGH 3 minutes, or until ham is heated through, turning after 1½ minutes. For each serving, place a ham slice on plate and spoon about ⅓ cup warm cherry mixture over top.

HINT:
A 3-ounce slice of ham is usually ⅓ inch thick.

Each serving equals:

DIABETIC: 2 Meat • 1 Fruit
138 Calories • 3 gm Fat • 15 gm Protein • 13 gm Carbohydrate • 855 mg Sodium • 1 gm Fiber
HE: 2 Protein • ⅔ Fruit • ¼ Slider

Ham Tetrazzini ✳

This is an updated version of a true 1950s favorite. The addition of the extra-lean ham provides just the right touch for this creamy dish.

✌ Serves 6 (1 cup)

> *1 full cup (6 ounces) diced Dubuque 97% fat-free ham or any extra-lean ham*
> *¹/₂ cup chopped onion*
> *1 (10 ³/₄-ounce) can Healthy Request Cream of Mushroom Soup*
> *³/₄ cup (3 ounces) shredded Kraft reduced-fat Cheddar cheese*
> *1 cup frozen peas*
> *2 tablespoons canned chopped pimiento*
> *2 tablespoons chopped fresh parsley or 2 teaspoons dried parsley flakes*
> *¹/₈ teaspoon black pepper*
> *2 cups chopped cooked spaghetti, rinsed and drained*

In a large skillet sprayed with butter-flavored cooking spray, sauté ham and onion until onion is tender, about 5 minutes. Stir in mushroom soup and Cheddar cheese. Cook over low heat, stirring often, until cheese melts. Add peas, pimiento, parsley, black pepper, and spaghetti. Mix well to combine. Lower heat and simmer 5 to 10 minutes, stirring often.

HINT:

1½ cups uncooked spaghetti usually cook to about 2 cups.

Each serving equals:

DIABETIC: 1½ Meat • 1½ Starch

197 Calories • 5 gm Fat • 15 gm Protein • 23 gm Carbohydrate • 669 mg Sodium • 1 gm Fiber

HE: 1⅓ Protein • 1 Bread • ¼ Vegetable • ¼ Slider • 8 Optional Calories

Macaroni and Cheese with Ham   ✳

This is true "comfort food" — made healthier. Enjoy!

✌ Serves 6

> 1½ cups (one 12-fluid-ounce can) Carnation Evaporated Skim Milk
> 3 tablespoons all-purpose flour
> 1½ cups (6 ounces) shredded Kraft reduced-fat Cheddar cheese
> 2 teaspoons prepared mustard
> ¼ teaspoon black pepper
> 2½ cups cooked elbow macaroni, rinsed and drained
> 1 full cup (6 ounces) diced Dubuque 97% fat-free ham or any extra-lean ham
> 3 tablespoons (¾ ounce) dried fine bread crumbs

Preheat oven to 350 degrees. Spray an 8-by-8-inch baking dish with butter-flavored cooking spray. In a covered jar, combine evaporated skim milk and flour. Shake well to combine. Pour milk mixture into a medium saucepan sprayed with butter-flavored cooking spray. Cook over medium heat, stirring often, until mixture starts to thicken. Stir in Cheddar cheese, mustard, and black pepper. Continue cooking, stirring often, until cheese melts. Add macaroni and ham. Mix well to combine. Pour mixture into prepared baking dish. Evenly sprinkle bread crumbs over top.

Quickly spray crumbs with butter-flavored cooking spray. Bake 30 minutes. Place baking dish on a wire rack and let set 5 minutes. Divide into 6 servings.

HINT:
  2 cups uncooked macaroni usually cook to about 2$\frac{1}{2}$ cups.

Each serving equals:

DIABETIC: 2 Meat • 1$\frac{1}{2}$ Starch • $\frac{1}{2}$ Skim Milk
258 Calories • 6 gm Fat • 21 gm Protein • 30 gm Carbohydrate • 560 mg Sodium • 1 gm Fiber
HE: 2 Protein • 1 Bread • $\frac{1}{2}$ Skim Milk

Deviled Ham on Noodles ✳

You'll be called an angel by anyone who shares this dish with you. It's downright heavenly!

✌ Serves 4

1/2 cup chopped onion
1³/4 cups (one 15-ounce can) Hunt's Chunky
   Tomato Sauce
2 tablespoons prepared mustard
1 tablespoon Brown Sugar Twin
1 full cup (6 ounces) diced Dubuque 97% fat-free
   ham or any extra-lean ham
2 cups hot cooked noodles, rinsed and drained

In a medium saucepan sprayed with butter-flavored cooking spray, sauté onion until tender, about 5 minutes. Add tomato sauce, mustard, and Brown Sugar Twin. Mix well to combine. Stir in ham. Lower heat. Simmer 10 minutes, stirring occasionally. For each serving, place 1/2 cup noodles on a plate and top with 1/2 cup ham mixture.

HINT:
  Full 1³/4 cups uncooked noodles usually cook to
    about 2 cups.

Each serving equals:

DIABETIC: 1¹/2 Starch • 1 Vegetable • 1 Meat
187 Calories • 3 gm Fat • 12 gm Protein • 28 gm Carbohydrate • 965 mg Sodium • 2 gm Fiber
HE: 2 Vegetable • 1 Bread • 1 Protein

Emerald Isle Ham Casserole ✳

A "jewel" of an Irish dish if there ever was one! You don't have to be of "the auld sod" to love this casserole.

✌ Serves 6

>3 cups shredded cabbage
>1 cup shredded carrots
>1³/₄ cups (3 ounces) uncooked noodles
>2 cups water
>1¹/₂ cups (one 12-fluid-ounce can) Carnation Evaporated Skim Milk
>3 tablespoons all-purpose flour
>¹/₈ teaspoon black pepper
>³/₄ cup (3 ounces) shredded Kraft reduced-fat Cheddar cheese
>¹/₂ cup (one 2.5-ounce jar) sliced mushrooms, drained
>1¹/₂ cups (9 ounces) diced Dubuque 97% fat-free ham or any extra-lean ham
>3 tablespoons (³/₄ ounce) dried fine bread crumbs

Preheat oven to 350 degrees. Spray an 8-by-8-inch baking dish with butter-flavored cooking spray. In a large saucepan, cook cabbage, carrots, and noodles in water until tender, about 10 to 12 minutes. Meanwhile, in a covered jar, combine evaporated skim milk, flour, and black pepper. Shake well to combine. Pour milk mixture into a large saucepan sprayed with butter-flavored cooking spray. Cook over medium heat, stirring often, until mixture starts to thicken. Add Cheddar cheese, mushrooms, and ham. Mix well to combine. Continue cooking, stirring constantly, until cheese melts. Drain cabbage mixture and stir in ham mixture. Mix gently to combine. Pour mixture into prepared baking dish. Sprinkle bread crumbs evenly over top. Quickly spray crumbs with butter-flavored cooking spray. Bake 20 to 25 minutes. Place baking dish on a wire rack and let set 5 minutes. Cut into 6 servings.

Each serving equals:

DIABETIC: 2 Meat • 1 Vegetable • 1 Starch • ½ Skim Milk

220 Calories • 4 gm Fat • 19 gm Protein • 27 gm Carbohydrate • 641 mg Sodium • 2 gm Fiber

HE: 1⅔ Protein • 1½ Vegetable • 1 Bread • ½ Skim Milk

Ham Casserole with Corn Topping ✳

Here's an unusual way I devised to moisten the biscuit mix. The ladies helping me mail out the newsletter really enjoyed tasting and testing it.

✌ Serves 6

1¹/₂ cups (one 12-fluid-ounce can) Carnation
    Evaporated Skim Milk
3 tablespoons all-purpose flour
¹/₂ cup (one 2.5-ounce jar) sliced mushrooms,
    drained
2 cups (one 16-ounce can) cut green beans, rinsed
    and drained
¹/₂ cup chopped onion
1 full cup (6 ounces) diced Dubuque 97% fat-free
    ham or any extra-lean ham
¹/₈ teaspoon black pepper
1 cup (one 8-ounce can) cream-style corn
³/₄ cup Bisquick Reduced Fat Baking Mix

Preheat oven to 350 degrees. Spray an 8-by-8-inch baking dish with butter-flavored cooking spray. In a covered jar, combine evaporated skim milk and flour. Shake well to combine. Pour milk mixture into a large skillet sprayed with butter-flavored cooking spray. Add mushrooms. Mix well to combine. Cook over medium heat, stirring often, until mixture starts to thicken. Stir in green beans, onion, ham, and black pepper. Spread mixture evenly into prepared baking dish. Bake

15 minutes. In a medium bowl, combine cream-style corn and baking mix. Drop corn mixture by spoonfuls to form 6 mounds evenly over partially baked ham mixture. Bake an additional 20 minutes or until mounds start to brown. Place baking dish on a wire rack and let set 5 minutes. Cut into 6 servings.

Each serving equals:

DIABETIC: 1 Vegetable • 1 Meat • 1 Starch • ½ Skim Milk

207 Calories • 3 gm Fat • 13 gm Protein • 32 gm Carbohydrate • 657 mg Sodium • 2 gm Fiber

HE: 1 Vegetable • 1 Bread • ⅔ Protein • ½ Skim Milk • 15 Optional Calories

Swiss, Ham, and Green Bean Shepherd's Pie ✳

Remember shepherd's pie, that cozy dish that's usually ground beef covered with mashed potatoes and baked to a golden goodness? Give my updated version a chance — I think you will be glad you did. (My son, Tommy, was!)

✌ Serves 4

1 full cup (6 ounces) diced Dubuque 97% fat-free ham or any extra-lean ham
1½ cups (one 12-fluid-ounce can) Carnation Evaporated Skim Milk
3 tablespoons all-purpose flour
½ cup (one 2.5-ounce jar) sliced mushrooms, drained
2 cups (one 16-ounce can) French style green beans, rinsed and drained
3 (¾-ounce) slices Kraft reduced-fat Swiss cheese, shredded
1⅔ cups water
1⅓ cups (3 ounces) instant potato flakes
⅓ cup Carnation Nonfat Dry Milk Powder
1 teaspoon dried parsley flakes
¼ teaspoon black pepper

Preheat oven to 350 degrees. Spray an 8-by-8-inch baking dish with butter-flavored cooking spray. In a large skillet sprayed with butter-flavored cooking spray, sauté ham for 3 to 4 minutes. Meanwhile, in a covered jar, combine evaporated skim milk and flour. Shake well to combine. Pour milk mixture into skillet with ham. Continue cooking, stirring constantly, until mixture thickens. Add mushrooms and green beans. Mix well to combine. Pour ham mixture into prepared baking dish. Evenly sprinkle Swiss cheese over top. Set aside. In a medium saucepan, bring water to a boil. Remove from heat. Stir in potato flakes, dry milk powder, parsley flakes, and black pepper. Fluff gently with a fork. Drop potato mixture by spoonfuls to form 4 mounds evenly over cheese. Bake 20 to 25 minutes. Place baking dish on a wire rack and let set 2 to 3 minutes. Cut into 4 servings.

Each serving equals:

DIABETIC: 1½ Meat • 1½ Starch • 1 Vegetable • 1 Skim Milk

308 Calories • 6 gm Fat • 23 gm Protein • 41 gm Carbohydrate • 908 mg Sodium • 2 gm Fiber

HE: 1¾ Protein • 1¼ Bread • 1¼ Vegetable • 1 Skim Milk

Corned Beef Pizza ✳

You may wonder about this pizza combination, but if you like corned beef (I do!), please give it a try. It's so good!

✌ Serves 12

> 1 (8-ounce) can Pillsbury refrigerated crescent dinner rolls
> 2 (2.5-ounce) packages Carl Buddig 90% lean corned beef, shredded
> $^1/_2$ cup chopped onion
> $2^1/_2$ cups purchased coleslaw mix
> 1 cup chunky salsa
> 2 tablespoons sloppy joe seasoning mix
> 1 (8-ounce) package Philadelphia Fat Free Cream Cheese
> $^1/_3$ cup Kraft Fat Free Thousand Island Dressing
> $^3/_4$ cup (3 ounces) shredded Kraft reduced-fat Cheddar cheese

Preheat oven to 450 degrees. Spray a rimmed 9-by-13-inch cookie sheet with butter-flavored cooking spray. Pat rolls into prepared pan, being sure to seal perforations. Bake 5 to 7 minutes or until light golden brown. Place cookie sheet on wire rack and allow to cool. In a large skillet sprayed with butter-flavored cooking spray, sauté corned beef, onion, and coleslaw mix until cabbage is tender, about 5 minutes. Add salsa and sloppy joe seasoning mix. Mix well to combine.

Simmer 5 minutes, stirring occasionally. In a medium bowl, stir cream cheese with a spoon until soft. Add Thousand Island dressing. Mix well to combine. Spread cream cheese mixture evenly over cooled crust. Layer cabbage mixture over cream cheese mixture. Sprinkle Cheddar cheese evenly over top. Return to oven. Continue baking 3 to 5 minutes or until cheese starts to melt. Place cookie sheet on a wire rack and let set 2 to 3 minutes. Cut into 12 servings.

HINT:
  2 cups shredded cabbage and ½ cup shredded carrots can be used in place of purchased coleslaw mix.

Each serving equals:

DIABETIC: 1 Meat • 1 Vegetable • ½ Starch • ½ Fat

129 Calories • 5 gm Fat • 8 gm Protein • 13 gm Carbohydrate • 537 mg Sodium • 1 gm Fiber

HE: 1 Protein • ⅔ Bread • ⅔ Vegetable • 13 Optional Calories

Reuben Pockets

So many people want quick and healthy sandwich recipes to take to work or school for their lunches. This was originally created with that need in mind. But you may want to try it even if you aren't planning to pack a lunch.

☙ Serves 4

2 (2.5-ounce) packages Carl Buddig 90% lean corned beef, finely shredded
³/₄ cup finely shredded lettuce
3 (³/₄-ounce) slices Kraft reduced-fat Swiss cheese, shredded
¹/₃ cup Kraft Fat Free Thousand Island Dressing
¹/₄ cup dill pickle relish
2 pita bread rounds, halved

In a medium bowl, combine corned beef, lettuce, and Swiss cheese. In a small bowl, combine Thousand Island dressing and dill pickle relish. Add dressing mixture to corned-beef mixture. Toss well to combine. Stuff each pita half with about ¹/₂ cup corned-beef mixture. Serve at once or cover and refrigerate until ready to serve.

HINT:
   To make opening pita rounds easier, place pita halves on a paper towel and microwave on HIGH 10 seconds. Remove and gently press open.

Each serving equals:

DIABETIC: 2 Meat • 1¹/₂ Starch

236 Calories • 8 gm Fat • 14 gm Protein • 27 gm Carbohydrate • 1,288 mg Sodium • 1 gm Fiber

HE: 2¹/₄ Protein • 1 Bread • ¹/₂ Vegetable • ¹/₄ Slider • 1 Optional Calorie

Kielbasa-Rice Casserole ✳

Come to the table hungry and walk away satisfied with this filling dish. I know my family appreciates that lean versions of our favorite deli meats are now widely available — so will yours.

✌ Serves 6

> *2 cups cooked rice*
> *1 cup frozen peas*
> *8 ounces Healthy Choice 97% lean kielbasa sausage, sliced into ¹/₄-inch pieces*
> *³/₄ cup (3 ounces) shredded Kraft reduced-fat Cheddar cheese*
> *1 tablespoon dried parsley flakes*
> *¹/₂ teaspoon lemon pepper*
> *1 (10 ³/₄-ounce) can Healthy Request Cream of Mushroom Soup*

Preheat oven to 350 degrees. Spray an 8-by-8-inch baking dish with butter-flavored cooking spray. In a large bowl, combine rice, peas, kielbasa sausage, and Cheddar cheese. Add parsley flakes, lemon pepper, and mushroom soup. Mix well to combine. Pour mixture into prepared baking dish. Bake 30 minutes. Place baking dish on a wire rack and let set 2 to 3 minutes. Cut into 6 servings.

HINTS:
1. 1¹/₃ cups uncooked rice usually cook to about 2 cups.

2. If you can't find Healthy Choice kielbasa sausage, use Healthy Choice frankfurters.

Each serving equals:

DIABETIC: 1½ Meat • 1½ Starch

175 Calories • 5 gm Fat • 14 gm Protein • 19 gm Carbohydrate • 656 mg Sodium • 2 gm Fiber

HE: 1½ Protein • 1 Bread • ¼ Slider • 11 Optional Calories

Hot Dog Stir Fry Skillet ✳

This may sound strange, but just ask my Tommy — or one of your own kids! Mine thinks it's great.

✌ Serves 4 (1 cup)

8 ounces diced Healthy Choice 97% fat-free frankfurters
1 cup chopped green bell pepper
1 cup (one 8-ounce can) pineapple chunks, packed in fruit juice, drained and ¹/₄ cup juice reserved
2 tablespoons apricot spreadable fruit spread
2 tablespoons reduced-sodium soy sauce
2 cups hot cooked rice

In a large skillet sprayed with olive-flavored cooking spray, sauté frankfurters and green pepper until browned, about 5 to 7 minutes. Stir in pineapple. In a small bowl, combine reserved pineapple juice, apricot spreadable fruit, and soy sauce. Add fruit mixture to frankfurter mixture. Mix well to combine. Lower heat and simmer 5 minutes, stirring occasionally. For each serving, place ¹/₂ cup rice on a plate and spoon about 1 cup frankfurter mixture over top.

HINT:
   1¹/₃ cups uncooked rice usually cook to about 2 cups.

Each serving equals:

DIABETIC: 1½ Starch • 1 Meat • 1 Fruit

209 Calories • 1 gm Fat • 10 gm Protein • 40 gm Carbohydrate • 606 mg Sodium • 2 gm Fiber

HE: 1⅓ Protein • 1 Fruit • 1 Bread • ½ Vegetable

Baked Pork with Sweet Potatoes and Applesauce ✳

Don't turn the page without giving this one a try. I think you may be surprised by the delicious flavor and aroma. James said it reminded him of some of the great food he enjoyed when stationed in Germany with the Army.

✌ Serves 4

4 (3-ounce) lean pork cutlets or tenderloins
3 cups (16 ounces) raw sweet potatoes, cut into
    1/4-inch slices
2 cups unsweetened applesauce
1/2 teaspoon apple pie spice
1/4 cup Brown Sugar Twin

Preheat oven to 350 degrees. Spray an 8-by-8-inch baking dish with butter-flavored cooking spray. In a large skillet sprayed with butter-flavored cooking spray, brown pork on both sides. Place browned pork in prepared baking dish. Arrange sweet potato slices over pork. In a small bowl, combine applesauce, apple pie spice, and Brown Sugar Twin. Pour applesauce mixture evenly over sweet potatoes. Cover and bake 45 to 50 minutes or until sweet potatoes are tender. Uncover and continue baking 10 minutes. Place baking dish on a wire rack and let set 5 minutes. Divide into 4 servings.

HINTS:
1. ¼ cup raisins can be added to applesauce.
2. Don't overbrown pork or it will become tough.

Each serving equals:

DIABETIC: 2 Meat • 1 Fruit • 1 Starch

313 Calories • 9 gm Fat • 23 gm Protein • 35 gm Carbohydrate • 64 mg Sodium • 3 gm Fiber

HE: 2¼ Protein • 1 Fruit • 1 Bread • 5 Optional Calories

Applesauce Pork Balls

※

This tasty dish really made a big hit with both Cliff and my daughter-in-law, Pam. I loved it too. Three out of three isn't bad, is it?

✌ Serves 6

> 16 ounces ground 90% lean pork
> 3/4 cup unsweetened applesauce
> 6 tablespoons (1 1/2 ounces) dried fine bread crumbs
> 1 teaspoon dried parsley flakes
> 1 3/4 cups (one 15-ounce can) Hunt's Chunky
>   Tomato Sauce
> 1/2 cup finely chopped onion
> 1 tablespoon Brown Sugar Twin

Preheat oven to 350 degrees. Spray an 8-by-8-inch baking dish with butter-flavored cooking spray. In a medium bowl, combine pork, applesauce, bread crumbs, and parsley flakes. Mix well with hands to combine. Form into twelve (1 1/2-inch) balls. Place balls in prepared baking dish. In a small bowl, combine tomato sauce, onion, and Brown Sugar Twin. Pour sauce mixture evenly over meatballs. Cover and bake 45 minutes. Uncover and continue baking 15 minutes. Place baking dish on a wire rack and let set 5 minutes. Divide into 6 servings.

Each serving equals:

DIABETIC: 2 Meat • 1 Starch

195 Calories • 7 gm Fat • 18 gm Protein • 15 gm Carbohydrate • 502 mg Sodium • 1 gm Fiber

HE: 2 Protein • 1$^1/_3$ Vegetable • $^1/_3$ Bread • $^1/_4$ Fruit • 1 Optional Calorie

Bavarian Casserole ✳

You don't have to wait for October to enjoy an Oktoberfest type of recipe. This is just as scrumptious any month of the year.

✌ Serves 6

> 16 ounces ground 90% lean pork
> $^3/_4$ cup chopped onion
> $1^3/_4$ cups (one $14^1/_2$-ounce can) Frank's Bavarian-style sauerkraut, undrained
> $^2/_3$ cup (2 ounces) uncooked regular rice
> $1^3/_4$ cups (one 15-ounce can) Hunt's Chunky Tomato Sauce
> $^1/_4$ teaspoon black pepper

Preheat oven to 350 degrees. Spray a 9-by-13-inch baking dish with butter-flavored cooking spray. In a large skillet sprayed with butter-flavored cooking spray, brown pork and onion. Stir in undrained sauerkraut, rice, tomato sauce, and black pepper. Mix well to combine. Pour mixture into prepared baking dish. Cover and bake 50 minutes. Uncover and continue baking 15 minutes. Place baking dish on a wire rack and let set 5 minutes. Divide into 6 servings.

HINT:

If you can't find Bavarian sauerkraut, use regular sauerkraut, $^1/_2$ teaspoon caraway seeds, and 1 teaspoon Brown Sugar Twin.

Each serving equals:

DIABETIC: 2 Meat • 2 Vegetable • ½ Starch

176 Calories • 4 gm Fat • 18 gm Protein • 17 gm Carbohydrate • 955 mg Sodium • 2 gm Fiber

HE: 2 Protein • 2 Vegetable • ⅓ Bread

Family Reunion Porkburgers ✳

I created this to share at my First Healthy Exchanges Potluck Family Reunion. It became an instant hit! As many of you can't come to DeWitt for our biannual reunion, I'm sharing the recipe with you. If you can't be with us in body, you can at least be here in spirit. Enjoy!

✌ Serves 8

> 16 ounces ground 90% lean pork
> 1/2 cup finely chopped onion
> 1 3/4 cups (one 15-ounce can) Hunt's Chunky Tomato Sauce
> 2 tablespoons Brown Sugar Twin
> 1 tablespoon vinegar
> 1 tablespoon Worcestershire sauce
> 1/4 cup grape spreadable fruit spread
> 1 tablespoon + 1 teaspoon all-purpose flour
> 8 reduced-calorie hamburger buns

In a large skillet sprayed with butter-flavored cooking spray, brown pork and onion. In a medium bowl, combine tomato sauce, Brown Sugar Twin, vinegar, Worcestershire sauce, grape spreadable fruit, and flour. Mix well to combine. Stir sauce mixture into meat mixture. Lower heat and simmer 15 to 20 minutes, stirring occasionally. For each serving, spoon about 1/2 cup meat mixture between a hamburger bun.

Each serving equals:

DIABETIC: 1¹/₂ Meat • 1 Starch • 1 Vegetable • ¹/₂ Fruit

211 Calories • 7 gm Fat • 10 gm Protein • 27 gm Carbohydrate • 513 mg Sodium • 2 gm Fiber

HE: 1¹/₂ Protein • 1 Bread • 1 Vegetable • ¹/₂ Fruit • 7 Optional Calories

Busy Man's Skillet

*

This is a recipe I created for my son Tom to take with him when he started living on his own with two other guys at the University of Iowa. He said to tell you it's both easy to prepare and good enough to invite the neighbors over.

Serves 4 (1 cup)

> 8 ounces ground 90% lean turkey or beef
> ½ cup chopped onion
> 1 cup (one 8-ounce can) Hunt's Tomato Sauce
> 1 cup frozen whole kernel corn
> 1 cup cooked spaghetti, rinsed and drained
> 1 teaspoon dried parsley flakes
> ⅛ teaspoon black pepper

In a large skillet sprayed with butter-flavored cooking spray, brown meat and onion. Add tomato sauce, corn, spaghetti, parsley flakes, and black pepper. Mix well to combine. Lower heat and simmer 5 to 10 minutes, stirring occasionally.

Hint:
> ¾ cup broken uncooked spaghetti usually cooks to about 1 cup.

Each serving equals:

DIABETIC: 2 Meat • 1 Vegetable • 1 Starch
197 Calories • 5 gm Fat • 14 gm Protein • 24 gm Carbohydrate • 427 mg Sodium • 3 gm Fiber
HE: 1½ Protein • 1¼ Vegetable • 1 Bread

Chili-Noodle Skillet Dinner ✳

This dish has all the sizzle of the Southwest. Even if it's below freezing outside, you can dine in on those sunny flavors.

✌ Serves 4 (1 cup)

> *8 ounces ground 90% lean turkey or beef*
> *¹/₄ cup chopped onion*
> *1³/₄ cups (one 14¹/₂-ounce can) stewed tomatoes, undrained*
> *2 teaspoons chili seasoning mix*
> *2 cups cooked noodles, rinsed and drained*

In a large skillet sprayed with olive-flavored cooking spray, brown meat and onion. Add undrained stewed tomatoes, chili seasoning mix, and noodles. Lower heat and simmer 10 minutes, stirring occasionally.

HINT:
> 1³/₄ cups uncooked noodles usually cook to about 2 cups.

Each serving equals:

DIABETIC: 2 Vegetable • 1¹/₂ Meat • 1 Starch
221 Calories • 6 gm Fat • 15 gm Protein • 27 gm Carbohydrate • 374 mg Sodium • 1 gm Fiber
HE: 1¹/₂ Protein • 1 Vegetable • 1 Bread

Special Spaghetti ✳

I created this while Tommy was home from college. He insisted on taking the recipe back to school with him. How often does that happen?

✌ Serves 4 (1 cup)

8 ounces ground 90% lean turkey or beef
1/2 cup chopped onion
1 3/4 cups (one 15-ounce can) Hunt's Chunky Tomato Sauce
1 teaspoon Italian seasoning
1 tablespoon Sugar Twin or Sprinkle Sweet
1 (10 3/4-ounce) can Healthy Request Cream of Mushroom Soup
2 cups cooked spaghetti, rinsed and drained
1/4 cup (3/4 ounce) grated Kraft fat-free Parmesan cheese

In a large skillet sprayed with olive-flavored cooking spray, brown meat and onion. Add tomato sauce, Italian seasoning, and Sugar Twin. Mix well to combine. Stir in mushroom soup. Lower heat. Simmer 10 minutes. Add spaghetti. Mix well to combine. Continue simmering 5 minutes, stirring occasionally. Stir in Parmesan cheese. Serve at once.

HINT:
  1 1/2 cups uncooked spaghetti usually cook to about 2 cups.

Each serving equals:

DIABETIC: 2 Meat • 2 Vegetable • 1½ Starch
275 Calories • 7 gm Fat • 18 gm Protein • 35 gm
Carbohydrate • 975 mg Sodium • 2 gm Fiber
HE: 2 Vegetable • 1¾ Protein • 1 Bread • ½ Slider
• 3 Optional Calories

Stove-Top Goulash ✳

This is an updated version of a goulash my mother made when I was a young girl growing up in a small Iowa town. Just eating this brought back wonderful childhood memories.

✌ Serves 6 (1 cup)

8 ounces ground 90% lean turkey or beef
1/2 cup chopped onion
1/2 teaspoon dried minced garlic
1 cup frozen peas
1/2 cup (one 2.5-ounce jar) sliced mushrooms, drained
1 3/4 cups (one 15-ounce can) Hunt's Chunky Tomato Sauce
2 cups cooked noodles, rinsed and drained
1/2 teaspoon black pepper
2 teaspoons paprika
3/4 cup (3 ounces) shredded Kraft reduced-fat Cheddar cheese

In a large skillet sprayed with olive-flavored cooking spray, brown meat and onion. Add minced garlic, peas, mushrooms, tomato sauce, noodles, black pepper, and paprika. Mix well to combine. Stir in Cheddar cheese. Lower heat. Cover and simmer 5 minutes, stirring occasionally.

HINT:
   Full 1 3/4 cups uncooked noodles usually cook to about 2 cups.

316

Each serving equals:

DIABETIC: 2 Vegetable • 1½ Meat • 1 Starch

219 Calories • 7 gm Fat • 16 gm Protein • 23 gm Carbohydrate • 587 mg Sodium • 2 gm Fiber

HE: 1⅔ Protein • 1½ Vegetable • 1 Bread

Supper Pot Potluck ✳

On a day dedicated to shopping, just throw this together before you head out the door. Supper will be ready when you get home. Okay, I know city folk call it dinner, but it's still supper in the Lund household.

✌ Serves 6 (1¼ cups)

> *16 ounces ground 90% lean turkey or beef*
> *3 cups (15 ounces) sliced raw potatoes*
> *1½ cups chopped celery*
> *2 cups sliced carrots*
> *1 cup chopped onion*
> *1½ cups frozen peas*
> *2 teaspoons Italian seasoning*
> *1¾ cups (one 15-ounce can) Hunt's Chunky*
>   *Tomato Sauce*

In a large skillet sprayed with butter-flavored cooking spray, brown meat. Meanwhile, place potatoes, celery, carrots, and onion in Crock-Pot container. Sprinkle peas over top. Spoon browned meat over vegetables. Stir Italian seasoning into tomato sauce. Evenly pour sauce over meat. Cover. Cook on LOW 6 to 8 hours. Stir well just before serving.

Each serving equals:

DIABETIC: 2 Vegetable • 2 Meat • 1 Starch

258 Calories • 8 gm Fat • 18 gm Protein • 29 gm Carbohydrate • 559 mg Sodium • 4 gm Fiber

HE: 2⅔ Vegetable • 2 Protein • 1 Bread

Hamburger Milk Gravy à la Tommy

I can't believe how many people have written to tell me how glad they are that Tommy loves hamburger milk gravy–based recipes, because they do too. Tommy said he wasn't surprised — as president of the Hamburger Milk Gravy Fan Club, he could have told me.

✌ Serves 4

> 8 ounces ground 90% lean turkey or beef
> 2 cups skim milk
> 3 tablespoons all-purpose flour
> 1/2 cup (4 ounces) Philadelphia Fat Free Cream Cheese
> 1/2 cup (one 2.5-ounce jar) sliced mushrooms, drained
> 1/2 cup frozen peas, thawed
> 2 tablespoons canned chopped pimiento
> 1 teaspoon dried parsley flakes
> 1/4 teaspoon black pepper
> 2 English muffins, split and toasted

In a large skillet sprayed with butter-flavored cooking spray, brown meat. In a covered jar, combine skim milk and flour. Shake well to combine. Pour milk mixture into browned meat. Mix well to combine. Stir in cream cheese. Add mushrooms, peas, pimiento, parsley flakes, and black pepper. Mix well to combine. Continue cooking, stirring occasionally, until mixture thickens. For each serving, place 1 English muffin half on a plate and spoon scant 1 cup of gravy mixture over top.

Each serving equals:

DIABETIC: 2 Meat • 2 Starch • ½ Skim Milk
245 Calories • 5 gm Fat • 22 gm Protein • 28 gm Carbohydrate • 503 mg Sodium • 2 gm Fiber
HE: 2 Protein • 1½ Bread • ½ Skim Milk • ¼ Vegetable

Hamburger Milk Gravy Pot Pie ✳

Tommy was home from college for the holidays, so you know I had to come up with another variation of his all-time favorite. He gave this his seal of approval.

✌ Serves 6

16 ounces ground 90% lean turkey or beef
¹/₂ cup frozen peas
2 cups (one 16-ounce can) sliced carrots, rinsed
*   and drained*
2 cups skim milk
3 tablespoons all-purpose flour
1 (7.5-ounce) can Pillsbury refrigerated buttermilk
*   biscuits*

Preheat oven to 350 degrees. Spray an 8-by-8-inch baking dish with butter-flavored cooking spray. In a large skillet sprayed with butter-flavored cooking spray, brown meat. Stir in peas and carrots. In a covered jar, combine skim milk and flour. Shake well to combine. Add milk mixture to meat mixture. Cook over medium heat, stirring often, until mixture thickens. Pour meat mixture into prepared baking dish. Separate biscuits and cut each biscuit into 4 pieces. Evenly sprinkle biscuit pieces over top of meat mixture. Bake 15 minutes or until biscuits are golden brown. Remove from oven. Quickly spray biscuit pieces with butter-flavored cooking spray. Place baking dish on a wire rack and let set 5 minutes. Cut into 6 servings.

Each serving equals:

DIABETIC: 2 Meat • 1¹/₂ Starch • ¹/₂ Vegetable
264 Calories • 8 gm Fat • 20 gm Protein • 28 gm Carbohydrate • 438 mg Sodium • 3 gm Fiber
HE: 2 Protein • 1¹/₃ Bread • ¹/₃ Vegetable • ¹/₃ Skim Milk • 7 Optional Calories

Crazy Pizza ✳

I served this pizza casserole to my family and everyone went crazy over it. It's amazing what happens to those plain refrigerated biscuits when you close that oven door!

✌ Serves 6

> 8 ounces ground 90% lean turkey or beef
> ½ cup (one 2.5-ounce jar) sliced mushrooms, drained
> ½ cup chopped green bell pepper
> ½ cup chopped onion
> ⅓ cup (1½ ounces) sliced ripe olives
> 1¾ cups (one 15-ounce can) Hunt's Chunky Tomato Sauce
> 1 tablespoon Sugar Twin or Sprinkle Sweet
> 1 teaspoon Italian seasoning
> 1 (7.5-ounce) can Pillsbury refrigerated buttermilk biscuits
> ⅓ cup (1½ ounces) shredded Kraft reduced-fat Cheddar cheese
> ⅓ cup (1½ ounces) shredded Kraft reduced-fat mozzarella cheese

Preheat oven to 350 degrees. Spray an 8-by-8-inch baking dish with olive-flavored cooking spray. In a large skillet sprayed with olive-flavored cooking spray, brown meat. Add mushrooms, green pepper, onion, and olives. Mix well to combine. Stir in tomato sauce, Sugar Twin, and Italian seasoning. Remove skillet from heat. Separate biscuits and cut each biscuit into 4 pieces. Gently stir biscuit pieces into meat mixture. Pour mixture into prepared baking dish. Bake 20 minutes. Sprinkle shredded Cheddar and mozzarella cheese evenly over the top. Continue baking until cheese melts, about 10 minutes. Place baking dish on a wire rack and let set 5 minutes. Cut into 6 servings.

Each serving equals:

DIABETIC: 2 Vegetable • 1½ Meat • 1 Starch
215 Calories • 7 gm Fat • 14 gm Protein • 24 gm Carbohydrate • 1052 mg Sodium • 2 gm Fiber
HE: 1⅔ Vegetable • 1½ Protein • 1¼ Bread • ¼ Fat • 1 Optional Calorie

Rice Pizza   ✳

The rice makes a wonderful crust in this easy pizza dish. I know, I was a little surprised to learn that not all dough is created alike.

✌ Serves 6

3 cups cooked rice
2 eggs, beaten or equivalent in egg substitute
³/₄ cup (3 counces) shredded Kraft reduced-fat
mozzarella cheese ☆
8 ounces ground 90% lean turkey or beef
¹/₂ cup chopped onion
¹/₂ cup chopped green bell pepper
1³/₄ cups (one 15-ounce can) Hunt's Chunky
Tomato Sauce
2 teaspoons Italian seasoning
¹/₄ cup (³/₄ ounce) grated Kraft fat-free Parmesan
cheese

Preheat oven to 450 degrees. Spray a 12-inch pizza pan with olive-flavored cooking spray. In a medium bowl, combine rice, eggs, and ¹/₄ cup mozzarella cheese. Mix well to combine. Spread rice mixture evenly on prepared pizza pan. Bake 20 minutes. Meanwhile, in a large skillet sprayed with olive-flavored cooking spray, brown meat, onion, and green pepper. Remove from heat and set aside. In a small bowl, combine tomato sauce and Italian seasoning. Spread sauce mixture evenly over baked crust. Top with meat mixture.

Evenly sprinkle Parmesan cheese and remaining ½ cup mozzarella cheese over top. Bake additional 10 to 15 minutes. Place pan on a wire rack and let set 5 minutes. Cut into 6 pieces.

HINT:
   2 cups uncooked rice usually cook to about 3 cups.

Each serving equals:

DIABETIC: 2 Meat • 1 Vegetable • 1 Starch

227 Calories • 7 gm Fat • 17 gm Protein • 24 gm Carbohydrate • 719 mg Sodium • 1 gm Fiber

HE: 2 Protein (⅓ limited) • 1½ Vegetable • 1 Bread

Iowa Stuffed Peppers ✳

I know when most of you think of Iowa, you say, "That's where the tall corn grows." Well, it does. And when you try these tasty stuffed peppers, you just may consider moving to Iowa. After all, our state has been mistaken for Heaven more than once.

✌ Serves 4

> 4 large green bell peppers
> 2 cups boiling water
> 8 ounces ground 90% lean turkey or beef
> ½ cup chopped onion
> 1¾ cups (one 15-ounce can) Hunt's Chunky
>   Tomato Sauce
> 1½ cups frozen whole kernel corn
> 1 teaspoon chili seasoning mix
> 3 tablespoons (¾ ounce) dried fine bread crumbs ☆
> ¼ teaspoon black pepper

Preheat oven to 350 degrees. Spray an 8-by-8-inch baking dish with butter-flavored cooking spray. Cut tops off green peppers. Discard seeds and membrane. Place peppers in a medium saucepan with boiling water. Cook on medium-high for 5 minutes. Drain peppers well. Meanwhile, in a large skillet sprayed with olive-flavored cooking spray, brown meat and onion. Stir in tomato sauce, corn, chili seasoning mix, 1 tablespoon bread crumbs, and black pepper. Place peppers in prepared baking dish. Evenly spoon meat mixture into peppers. Sprinkle about ¹/₂ tablespoon bread crumbs over top of each. Quickly spray tops with butter-flavored cooking spray. Bake 30 minutes. Place baking dish on a wire rack and let set 5 minutes.

Each serving equals:

DIABETIC: 2 Vegetable • 1½ Meat • 1 Starch
239 Calories • 7 gm Fat • 15 gm Protein • 29 gm Carbohydrate • 714 mg Sodium • 4 gm Fiber
HE: 2¼ Vegetable • 1½ Protein • 1 Bread

Smothered "Steak and Onions" ✳

All the flavor of the real thing, but without the extra fat! If you've never lost your taste for this oh-so-good-but-not-so-good-for-you dish, here's the answer — and it's a winner.

✌ Serves 6

16 ounces ground 90% lean turkey or beef
¼ teaspoon black pepper
1¾ cups (one 14½-ounce can) beef broth ☆
6 tablespoons (1½ ounces) dried fine bread crumbs
2 cups sliced onion
3 tablespoons all-purpose flour

In a large bowl, combine meat, black pepper, ¼ cup beef broth, and bread crumbs. Mix well with hands to combine. Using a ⅓-cup measure as a guide, form 6 patties. Place patties in a large skillet sprayed with butter-flavored cooking spray and brown on both sides. Layer onion evenly over browned patties. In a covered jar, combine remaining 1½ cups beef broth and flour. Shake well to combine. Pour broth mixture evenly over onion. Lower heat. Cover and simmer 20 to 25 minutes. For each serving, place 1 patty on plate and evenly spoon onion sauce over top.

Each serving equals:

DIABETIC: 2 Meat • ¹/₂ Vegetable • ¹/₂ Starch

179 Calories • 7 gm Fat • 16 gm Protein • 13 gm Carbohydrate • 384 mg Sodium • 1 gm Fiber

HE: 2 Protein • ²/₃ Vegetable • ¹/₂ Bread • 6 Optional Calories

Bayou Country Meat Loaf ✳

Cliff really enjoyed his job as "official taste tester" while I was experimenting with this recipe. It may get hot down there in Cajun country, but that only seems to encourage the appetite! It must be all those spicy spices. . . .

✌ Serves 6

16 ounces ground 90% lean turkey or beef
1 cup (one 8-ounce can) Hunt's Tomato Sauce ☆
1 cup cooked cold rice
¹/₄ cup chopped onion
2 to 4 drops Tabasco sauce
1³/₄ cups (one 14¹/₂-ounce can) stewed tomatoes,
* undrained*
1 teaspoon prepared mustard
1 tablespoon Sugar Twin or Sprinkle Sweet
1 teaspoon Cajun seasoning

Preheat oven to 350 degrees. Spray an 8-by-8-inch baking dish with butter-flavored cooking spray. In a large bowl, combine meat, ¹/₃ cup tomato sauce, rice, onion, and Tabasco sauce. Mix well with hands to combine. Pat meat mixture into prepared baking dish. Bake 30 minutes. In a medium bowl, combine remaining ²/₃ cup tomato sauce, undrained stewed tomatoes, mustard, Sugar Twin, and Cajun seasoning. Mix well to combine. Spoon tomato mixture evenly over meat loaf. Bake an additional 15 to 20 minutes.

Place baking dish on a wire rack and let set 10 minutes. Cut into 6 servings.

HINT:

²/₃ cup uncooked rice usually cooks to about 1 cup.

Each serving equals:

DIABETIC: 2 Meat • 1 Vegetable • ½ Starch

170 Calories • 6 gm Fat • 15 gm Protein • 14 gm Carbohydrate • 530 mg Sodium • 1 gm Fiber

HE: 2 Protein • 1⅓ Vegetable • ⅓ Bread • 1 Optional Calorie

Carrot Meat Loaf with Cheese Sauce

✳

Meat loaf is one of the best man-pleasing dishes I know — and I know quite a few of them by now. You'll be surprised at how much the carrots add to this succulent main dish.

✌ Serves 6

> 2 cups (one 16-ounce can) sliced carrots, rinsed and drained
> 16 ounces ground 90% lean turkey or beef
> 6 tablespoons (1¹/₂ ounces) dried fine bread crumbs
> ¹/₂ cup diced onion
> ¹/₂ teaspoon lemon pepper
> 1¹/₂ cups (one 12-fluid-ounce can) Carnation Evaporated Skim Milk ☆
> 3 tablespoons all-purpose flour
> ³/₄ cup (3 ounces) shredded Kraft reduced-fat Cheddar cheese
> ¹/₂ cup (one 2.5-ounce jar) sliced mushrooms, drained
> ¹/₄ teaspoon black pepper

Preheat oven to 375 degrees. Spray an 8-by-8-inch baking dish with butter-flavored cooking spray. In a large bowl, combine carrots, meat, bread crumbs, onion, lemon pepper, and ¹/₄ cup evaporated skim milk. Mix well with hands to combine. Pat meat mixture into prepared baking dish. Bake 55 to 60 minutes. Place baking dish on a wire rack and let set while preparing cheese sauce. In a covered jar, combine remaining $1\frac{1}{4}$ cups evaporated skim milk and flour. Shake well to combine. Pour milk mixture into a medium saucepan sprayed with butter-flavored cooking spray. Add Cheddar cheese, mushrooms, and black pepper. Cook over medium heat, stirring often, until mixture thickens and cheese melts. Pour hot cheese sauce over meat mixture. Let set 2 to 3 minutes. Cut into 6 servings.

Each serving equals:

DIABETIC: 3 Meat • 1 Starch • 1 Vegetable

257 Calories • 9 gm Fat • 24 gm Protein • 20 gm Carbohydrate • 384 mg Sodium • 2 gm Fiber

HE: $2\frac{2}{3}$ Protein • 1 Vegetable • $\frac{1}{2}$ Bread

Ranch Hand Meat Loaf ✳

After a hard day's work at school, the office, the factory, or the farm, this meat loaf will make everyone feel appreciated. The aroma as they walk in the door just says, "Welcome home!"

✌ Serves 6

1 cup (one 8-ounce can) Hunt's Tomato Sauce
¹/₄ cup Brown Sugar Twin
2 tablespoons vinegar
1 teaspoon prepared mustard
16 ounces ground 90% lean turkey or beef
12 small fat-free saltine crackers, crushed
¹/₄ teaspoon black pepper

Preheat oven to 350 degrees. Spray an 8-by-8-inch baking dish with butter-flavored cooking spray. In a medium saucepan, combine tomato sauce, Brown Sugar Twin, vinegar, and mustard. Cook over medium heat, stirring often, until mixture just comes to boil. Remove from heat. In a large bowl, combine meat, cracker crumbs, black pepper, and ¹/₄ cup of hot tomato sauce mixture. Mix well with hands to combine. Pat meat mixture into prepared baking dish. Pour remaining sauce evenly over top. Bake 45 to 50 minutes. Place baking dish on a wire rack and let set 5 minutes. Cut into 6 servings.

Each serving equals:

DIABETIC: 2 Meat • ¹/₂ Starch

151 Calories • 7 gm Fat • 14 gm Protein • 8 gm Carbohydrate • 412 mg Sodium • 1 gm Fiber

HE: 2 Protein • ³/₄ Vegetable • ¹/₃ Bread • 4 Optional Calories

Desserts

Rice-Raisin Pudding ✳

Celebrate old-fashioned flavor using modern ingredients. This tastes just like my favorite rice pudding when I was a girl.

✌ Serves 4

> 1 (4-serving) package JELL-O sugar-free vanilla cook & serve pudding mix
> 2 cups skim milk
> 1/2 cup raisins
> 2/3 cup (2 ounces) uncooked instant rice

In an 8-cup glass measuring bowl, combine dry pudding mix and skim milk. Mix well using a wire whisk. Stir in raisins and rice. Cover and microwave on HIGH (100% power) 6 to 7 minutes, stirring every 2 minutes. Place bowl on a wire rack and let set 2 to 3 minutes. Mix well. Evenly spoon mixture into 4 dessert dishes. Serve warm or cold.

Each serving equals:

DIABETIC: 1 Fruit • 1 Starch • 1/2 Skim Milk
168 Calories • 0 gm Fat • 6 gm Protein • 36 gm Carbohydrate • 207 mg Sodium • 1 gm Fiber
HE: 1 Fruit • 1/2 Bread • 1/2 Skim Milk • 1/4 Slider

Easy Lemon Pudding

Use this easy, fluffy pudding in any of your recipes that call for prepared instant lemon pudding. No one will know the difference.

✌ Serves 4

1 (4-serving) package JELL-O sugar-free lemon gelatin
1 (4-serving) package JELL-O sugar-free instant vanilla pudding mix
²/₃ cup Carnation Nonfat Dry Milk Powder
1¹/₂ cups water
¹/₂ cup Cool Whip Lite

In a large bowl, combine dry gelatin, dry pudding mix, and dry milk powder. Add water. Mix well using a wire whisk. Blend in Cool Whip Lite. Evenly spoon mixture into 4 dessert dishes. Refrigerate at least 10 minutes.

Each serving equals:

DIABETIC: ¹/₂ Skim Milk • ¹/₂ Starch

113 Calories • 1 gm Fat • 12 gm Protein • 14 gm Carbohydrate • 437 mg Sodium • 0 gm Fiber

HE: ¹/₂ Skim Milk • ¹/₂ Slider • 15 Optional Calories

Maple Custard

Maple trees all across America would be proud of this yummy custard created in their honor.

✌ Serves 4

> 1 (4-serving) package JELL-O sugar-free vanilla cook & serve pudding mix
> ²/₃ cup Carnation Nonfat Dry Milk Powder
> 1¹/₂ cups water
> ¹/₂ cup Cary's Sugar Free Maple Syrup
> ¹/₄ cup Cool Whip Lite

In an 8-cup glass measuring bowl, combine dry pudding mix and dry milk powder. Add water and maple syrup. Mix well using a wire whisk. Cover. Microwave on HIGH (100% power) 4 minutes, stirring after 2 minutes. Pour hot mixture into 4 dessert dishes. Refrigerate at least 1 hour. Just before serving, top each with 1 tablespoon Cool Whip Lite.

Each serving equals:

DIABETIC: 1 Starch

84 Calories • less than 1 gm Fat • 4 gm Protein • 16 gm Carbohydrate • 242 mg Sodium • 0 gm Fiber

HE: ¹/₄ Skim Milk • ¹/₂ Slider • 10 Optional Calories

Banana Pudding with Raspberry Sauce

If you want to impress your guests or simply show your family how special they are, serve this outstanding dessert. My staff, who by now have tasted just about everything imaginable, still rave about the day they enjoyed this spectacular treat.

✌ Serves 6

  1 (4-serving) package JELL-O sugar-free instant banana pudding mix
  2 cups skim milk
  2 cups (2 medium) sliced bananas
  1 (4-serving) package JELL-O sugar-free vanilla cook & serve pudding mix
  1 (4-serving) package JELL-O sugar-free raspberry gelatin
  1¹/₂ cups frozen unsweetened red raspberries, thawed and liquid reserved
  Water
  6 tablespoons Cool Whip Lite

In a medium bowl, combine dry instant pudding mix and skim milk. Mix well using a wire whisk. Add sliced bananas. Mix gently to combine. Evenly spoon pudding mixture into 6 dessert dishes. Refrigerate while preparing sauce. In a medium saucepan, combine dry cook-and-serve pudding mix and dry gelatin. Add enough water to reserved raspberry juice to make 1¹/₃ cups liquid. Add liquid to dry pudding mixture. Mix well to combine. Cook over medium heat, stirring constantly, until mixture thickens and starts to boil. Remove from heat. Gently stir in thawed raspberries. Place pan on a wire rack and allow to cool 30 minutes. Evenly drizzle about ¼ cup raspberry sauce over each dessert dish and top with 1 tablespoon Cool Whip Lite.

Each serving equals:

DIABETIC: 1 Fruit • ½ Skim Milk • ½ Starch

145 Calories • 1 gm Fat • 9 gm Protein • 25 gm Carbohydrate • 317 mg Sodium • 1 gm Fiber

HE: 1 Fruit • ⅓ Skim Milk • ½ Slider • 6 Optional Calories

Candy Treat Tapioca Pudding

Cliff said this was every bit as good as a candy bar. I don't know if I would go that far, but it sure seemed to satisfy my sweet tooth the day I stirred it up!

✌ Serves 4

1 (4-serving) package JELL-O sugar-free vanilla cook & serve pudding mix
2 cups skim milk
3 tablespoons quick tapioca
1/4 cup Brown Sugar Twin
1 tablespoon (1/4 ounce) mini chocolate chips
2 tablespoons (1/2 ounce) chopped dry-roasted peanuts
1/4 cup (1/2 ounce) miniature marshmallows
1/4 cup Cool Whip Lite

In a medium saucepan, combine dry pudding mix, skim milk, and dry tapioca. Let set 5 minutes. Stir in Brown Sugar Twin. Cook over medium heat, stirring often, until mixture thickens and starts to boil. Remove from heat. Place pan on a wire rack and allow to cool 15 minutes. Gently fold chocolate chips, peanuts, and marshmallows into pudding mixture. Evenly spoon mixture into 4 dessert dishes. Refrigerate at least 30 minutes. When serving, top each with 1 tablespoon Cool Whip Lite.

Each serving equals:

DIABETIC: 1 Starch • ½ Skim Milk • ½ Fat

140 Calories • 3 gm Fat • 5 gm Protein • 24 gm Carbohydrate • 212 mg Sodium • 0 gm Fiber

HE: ½ Skim Milk • ¼ Fat • ¾ Slider • 13 Optional Calories

Polynesian Fruit Dessert

This quick-to-fix and scrumptious-to-taste treat stirs up fast. It's like instant paradise in a dessert dish.

❧ Serves 4

1 cup (one 8-ounce can) crushed pineapple, packed in fruit juice, undrained
1 teaspoon coconut extract
³/₄ cup Yoplait plain fat-free yogurt
¹/₄ cup water
1 (4-serving) package JELL-O sugar-free instant vanilla pudding mix
1 cup (1 medium) sliced banana
1 cup (one 11-ounce can) mandarin oranges, rinsed and drained
2 teaspoons flaked coconut
2 maraschino cherries, halved

In a medium bowl, combine pineapple, coconut extract, yogurt, and water. Add dry pudding mix. Mix well using a wire whisk. Fold in banana and mandarin oranges. Spoon mixture evenly into 4 dessert dishes. Garnish each with ¹/₂ teaspoon coconut and ¹/₂ maraschino cherry. Refrigerate at least 10 minutes before serving.

Each serving equals:

DIABETIC: 2 Fruit *or* 1 Fruit • 1 Starch

141 Calories • less than 1 gm Fat • 3 gm Protein • 33 gm Carbohydrate • 428 mg Sodium • 2 gm Fiber

HE: 1½ Fruit • ¼ Skim Milk • ¼ Slider • 15 Optional Calories

Oatmeal-Raisin Cookies   ✳

Cliff loves cookies — really loves them — and he loves these cookies even more than I expected. Aren't these cozy treats everyone's favorite munchie?

✌ Serves 8 (3 each)

1¹/₂ cups (4³/₄ ounces) quick oats
¹/₂ cup + 1 tablespoon all-purpose flour
1 teaspoon baking powder
¹/₂ teaspoon baking soda
1 teaspoon pumpkin pie spice
2 tablespoons Brown Sugar Twin
¹/₃ cup Sugar Twin or Sprinkle Sweet
2 tablespoons + 2 teaspoons reduced-calorie
  margarine
1 egg, slightly beaten, or equivalent in egg substitute
¹/₂ cup unsweetened applesauce
¹/₄ cup Yoplait plain fat-free yogurt
6 tablespoons raisins

Preheat oven to 350 degrees. Spray 2 cookie sheets with butter-flavored cooking spray. In a large bowl, combine oats, flour, baking powder, baking soda, pumpkin pie spice, Brown Sugar Twin, and Sugar Twin. Melt margarine and blend into oats mixture. Add egg, applesauce, yogurt, and raisins. Mix gently to combine. Drop by tablespoon to form 24 cookies on prepared cookie sheets. Bake 20 to 22 minutes. Place cookie sheets on wire racks and allow to cool completely.

Each serving equals:

DIABETIC: 1 Starch • ½ Fruit • ½ Fat

111 Calories • 3 gm Fat • 3 gm Protein • 18 gm Carbohydrate • 148 mg Sodium • 3 gm Fiber

HE: 1⅓ Bread • ½ Fat • ½ Fruit • 19 Optional Calories

Jo's Sweetened Condensed Milk

I did it! Whenever I can create a healthy version of a purchased product, I call it cracking the code. Well, I figured out how to make sweetened condensed milk without fat or sugar. Here's how I did it:

> *¹/₂ cup cold water*
> *1¹/₃ cups Carnation Nonfat Dry Milk Powder*
> *¹/₂ cup Sugar Twin or Sprinkle Sweet*

Place cold water in a 2-cup glass measure. Stir in dry milk powder until mixture makes a smooth paste. Cover and microwave on **HIGH** (100% power) 45 to 60 seconds or until mixture is very hot, but not to the boiling point. Stir in Sugar Twin. Mix well to dissolve. Cover and refrigerate at least 2 hours before using.

Will keep up to two weeks in refrigerator. Use in any recipe that calls for sweetened condensed milk. Makes equivalent of one 12-fluid-ounce can of commercial brand.

Each recipe equals:

DIABETIC: 4 Skim Milk

366 Calories • 0 gm Fat • 32 gm Protein • 59 gm Carbohydrate • 520 mg Sodium • 0 gm Fiber

HE: 4 Skim Milk • ¹/₂ Slider • 4 Optional Calories

Graham Sensations ✳

Now that we've got a recipe for sweetened condensed milk (page 350), how about a cookie recipe using it in all its goodness?

✌ Serves 8 (3 each)

> 1¼ cups purchased graham cracker crumbs or 20 (2½-inch squares) made into crumbs
> ¼ cup all-purpose flour
> ¼ teaspoon salt
> 1 recipe Jo's Sweetened Condensed Milk
> 1 teaspoon vanilla extract
> 1 teaspoon coconut extract
> ¼ cup (1 ounce) chopped pecans
> ¼ cup (1 ounce) mini chocolate chips
> ¼ cup flaked coconut

Preheat oven to 350 degrees. Spray a cookie sheet with butter-flavored cooking spray. In a large bowl, combine graham cracker crumbs, flour, and salt. Make a well in center. Add Jo's Sweetened Condensed Milk and vanilla and coconut extracts. Mix until well blended. Stir in pecans, chocolate chips and coconut. Drop by teaspoonfuls onto prepared cookie sheet to form 24 balls. Bake 10 minutes. Place cookie sheet on a wire rack and allow to cool.

Each serving equals:

DIABETIC: 1½ Starch • ½ Skim Milk • 1 Fat

191 Calories • 6 gm Fat • 6 gm Protein • 29 gm Carbohydrate • 215 mg Sodium • 2 gm Fiber

HE: 1 Bread • ½ Skim Milk • ½ Fat • ¼ Slider • 14 Optional Calories

Strawberry Hill Shortcakes

I think if I knew I was eating my last meal ever, my dessert of choice would be this strawberry delight.

✌ Serves 4

> *3/4 cup Bisquick Reduced Fat Baking Mix*
> *1/3 cup Carnation Nonfat Dry Milk Powder*
> *1/3 cup + 2 tablespoons Sugar Twin or Sprinkle Sweet ☆*
> *2 tablespoons Kraft fat-free mayonnaise*
> *1/3 cup water*
> *4 cups sliced fresh strawberries ☆*
> *1/4 cup Cool Whip Lite*

Preheat oven to 415 degrees. Spray baking sheet with butter-flavored cooking spray. In a medium bowl, combine baking mix, dry milk powder, and 2 tablespoons Sugar Twin. Add mayonnaise and water. Mix well to combine. Drop by tablespoon onto prepared baking sheet to form 4 shortcakes. Bake 8 to 12 minutes or until golden brown. Place baking sheet on a wire rack and allow to cool. Meanwhile, in a medium bowl, mash 1 cup strawberries with a fork or potato masher. Add remaining 1/3 cup Sugar Twin. Mix well to combine. Stir in remaining 3 cups strawberries. Cover and refrigerate until ready to serve. For each serving, split shortcakes in half, place bottom half on a serving plate, spoon about 1/2 cup strawberry mixture over bottom, arrange top half over strawberries, spoon about ¼ cup strawberry mixture over top and garnish with 1 tablespoon Cool Whip Lite.

Each serving equals:

DIABETIC: 1 Starch • 1 Fruit

174 Calories • 3 gm Fat • 4 gm Protein • 33 gm Carbohydrate • 348 mg Sodium • 5 gm Fiber

HE: 1 Bread • 1 Fruit • ¼ Skim Milk • ¼ Slider • 3 Optional Calories

Cherry Swirl Coffee Cake　　　❋

As good as any cherry coffee cake in the land! No one would ever believe it's sugar free unless you told them, and then they still wouldn't believe you.

✌ Serves 8

> 1 (4-serving) package JELL-O sugar-free vanilla cook & serve pudding mix
> 1 (4-serving) package JELL-O sugar-free cherry gelatin
> 1^1/$_3$ cups water ✩
> 2 cups (one 16-ounce can) tart red cherries, packed in water, drained
> 1 teaspoon almond extract
> 1^1/$_2$ cups Bisquick Reduced Fat Baking Mix
> ^{1}/$_4$ cup Sugar Twin or Sprinkle Sweet
> ^{2}/$_3$ cup Carnation Nonfat Dry Milk Powder
> 1 tablespoon + 1 teaspoon reduced-calorie margarine, melted and slightly cooled
> 1 teaspoon vanilla extract
> 2 eggs, slightly beaten, or equivalent in egg substitute

Preheat oven to 350 degrees. Spray a 9-by-9-inch cake pan with butter-flavored cooking spray. In a medium saucepan, combine dry pudding mix, dry gelatin, 1 cup water, and cherries. Cook over medium heat, stirring constantly, until mixture thickens and starts to boil. Remove from heat.

Stir in almond extract. Place pan on a wire rack and allow to cool. Meanwhile, in a medium bowl, combine baking mix, Sugar Twin, and dry milk powder. In a small bowl, combine margarine, remaining $1/3$ cup water, vanilla extract, and eggs. Add liquid mixture to baking mix mixture. Mix well to combine. Spread $2/3$ of the batter into prepared cake pan. Evenly spread cherry mixture over batter. Drop remaining batter by teaspoon over cherry mixture to form 8 mounds. Bake 20 to 25 minutes or until light golden brown. Quickly spray top with butter-flavored cooking spray. Place cake pan on a wire rack and let set at least 5 minutes. Cut into 8 servings. Good warm or cold.

Each serving equals:

DIABETIC: 1 Starch • 1 Fruit

172 Calories • 4 gm Fat • 7 gm Protein • 27 gm Carbohydrate • 406 mg Sodium • 1 gm Fiber

HE: 1 Bread • $1/2$ Fruit • $1/2$ Skim Milk • $1/4$ Fat • $1/4$ Protein (limited) • 18 Optional Calories

Double Chocolate Cupcakes ✳

These cupcakes taste a lot like brownies. If you have any chocolate lovers in the house, this should quickly become their "best of the best!"

✌ Serves 12

1¹/₂ cups all-purpose flour
¹/₂ cup Sugar Twin or Sprinkle Sweet
¹/₄ cup unsweetened cocoa
1 teaspoon baking soda
¹/₂ teaspoon salt
¹/₂ cup unsweetened orange juice
¹/₃ cup water
3 tablespoons vegetable oil
1 tablespoon white vinegar
1 teaspoon vanilla extract
¹/₄ cup (1 ounce) mini chocolate chips

Preheat oven to 375 degrees. Spray a 12-cup muffin pan with butter-flavored cooking spray or line with paper liners. In a medium bowl, combine flour, Sugar Twin, cocoa, baking soda, and salt. Make a well in center of mixture. In a small bowl, combine orange juice, water, oil, vinegar, and vanilla extract. Add liquid mixture to dry ingredients, stirring just until moistened. Fold in chocolate chips. Fill prepared muffin cups ²/₃ full. Bake 12 minutes or until a toothpick inserted in center comes out clean. Remove from pan immediately and allow to cool on a wire rack.

Each serving equals:

DIABETIC: 1 Starch • 1 Fat

108 Calories • 4 gm Fat • 2 gm Protein • 16 gm Carbohydrate • 197 mg Sodium • 1 gm Fiber

HE: ³/₄ Fat • ²/₃ Bread • ¹/₄ Slider • 7 Optional Calories

French Pear Cream Dessert

It's quick, it's colorful, and it looks and tastes as if you really fussed. That's my formula for a great meal-ender!

✌ Serves 8

12 (2¹/₂-inch square) graham crackers ☆
2 cups (one 16-ounce can) pear halves, packed in fruit juice, drained and liquid reserved
1 (4-serving) package JELL-O sugar-free instant vanilla pudding mix
²/₃ cup Carnation Nonfat Dry Milk Powder
Water
¹/₂ teaspoon brandy extract
¹/₄ cup raspberry spreadable fruit spread
1 cup Cool Whip Lite ☆

Evenly arrange 9 of the graham crackers in a 9-by-9-inch cake pan. Coarsely chop pears and evenly sprinkle over graham crackers. In a medium bowl, combine dry pudding mix and dry milk powder. Add enough water to reserved pear juice to make 1 cup liquid. Add liquid to pudding mixture. Mix well using a wire whisk. Blend in brandy extract, raspberry spreadable fruit, and ¹/₄ cup Cool Whip Lite. Spread pudding mixture evenly over pears. Refrigerate 30 minutes. Spread remaining ³/₄ cup Cool Whip Lite evenly over filling. Crush remaining 3 graham crackers. Sprinkle crumbs evenly over the top. Cover and refrigerate at least 2 hours. Cut into 8 servings.

Each serving equals:

DIABETIC: 1 Fruit • 1 Starch

149 Calories • 2 gm Fat • 3 gm Protein • 30 gm Carbohydrate • 264 mg Sodium • 1 gm Fiber

HE: 1 Fruit • ½ Bread • ¼ Skim Milk • ¼ Slider • 12 Optional Calories

Butter Brickle Dessert ✳

This elegant, crunchy dessert is so easy that you'll want to make it often. The coconut extract will make you think I had you open a whole package of coconut and throw it in, but I didn't! It just tastes that way.

✌ Serves 8

> 12 (2¹/₂-inch square) graham crackers ☆
> 1 (4-serving) package JELL-O sugar-free instant
>   butterscotch pudding mix
> ²/₃ cup Carnation Nonfat Dry Milk Powder
> 1²/₃ cups water
> ¹/₄ cup (1 ounce) chopped pecans ☆
> 3 tablespoons flaked coconut ☆
> 1 teaspoon coconut extract
> 1 cup Cool Whip Lite

Evenly arrange 9 of the graham crackers in a 9-by-9-inch cake pan. In a large bowl, combine dry pudding mix and dry milk powder. Add water. Mix well using a wire whisk. Stir in 3 tablespoons pecans, 2 tablespoons flaked coconut, and coconut extract. Pour pudding mixture evenly over graham crackers. Cover and refrigerate 1 hour. Just before serving, spread Cool Whip Lite evenly over pudding mixture. Crush remaining 3 graham cracker squares into crumbs. In a small bowl, combine graham cracker crumbs, remaining 1 tablespoon pecans, and remaining 1 tablespoon flaked coconut. Sprinkle crumb mixture evenly over top of dessert. Cut into 8 servings.

Each serving equals:

DIABETIC: 1 Starch • 1 Fat

129 Calories • 5 gm Fat • 3 gm Protein • 18 gm Carbohydrate • 264 mg Sodium • 1 gm Fiber

HE: ½ Fat • ½ Bread • ¼ Skim Milk • ¼ Slider • 18 Optional Calories

Cholocate Eclair Dessert ✳

You'll find this dessert quickly becomes a family favorite. It just tastes so good, they'll think it's got to be bad, but guess what . . . it's good for you, too!

✌ Serves 12

36 (2¹/₂-inch) graham cracker squares
2 (4-serving) packages JELL-O sugar-free instant vanilla pudding mix
2 cups Carnation Nonfat Dry Milk Powder ☆
4¹/₄ cups water ☆
1¹/₂ cups Cool Whip Lite ☆
2 teaspoons vanilla extract ☆
1 (4-serving) package JELL-O sugar-free instant chocolate pudding mix
1 tablespoon chocolate syrup

Evenly arrange 12 graham crackers in a 9-by-13-inch cake pan. In a large bowl, combine dry vanilla pudding mixes, 1¹/₃ cups dry milk powder, and 3 cups water. Mix well using a wire whisk. Blend in ¹/₂ cup Cool Whip Lite and 1 teaspoon vanilla extract. Mix gently to combine. Spread half of pudding mixture evenly over graham crackers. Layer another 12 graham crackers over top. Evenly spread remaining pudding mixture over graham crackers. Top with remaining 12 graham crackers. In a medium bowl, combine dry chocolate pudding mix, remaining ²/₃ cup dry milk powder, remaining 1 teaspoon vanilla extract and remaining 1¼ cups water. Mix well using a wire whisk. Spread chocolate mixture evenly over top of graham crackers. Cover and refrigerate at least 1 hour. Just before serving, spread remaining 1 cup Cool Whip Lite evenly over top. Drizzle chocolate syrup evenly over Cool Whip Lite. Refrigerate at least 1 hour. Cut into 12 servings.

HINT:
Best if made the night before.

Each serving equals:

DIABETIC: 1½ Starch • ½ Skim Milk • ½ Fat
179 Calories • 3 gm Fat • 6 gm Protein • 32 gm Carbohydrate • 519 mg Sodium • 1 gm Fiber
HE: 1 Bread • ½ Skim Milk • ½ Slider • 8 Optional Calories

Cherry-Pineapple Dessert Bars ✳

This is a great one to bring to bake sales or potluck parties — speedy to prepare, and a crowd-pleaser for anyone from eight to eighty.

✌ Serves 12

1 (8-ounce) can Pillsbury refrigerated crescent dinner rolls
1 (8-ounce) package Philadelphia Fat Free Cream Cheese
Sugar substitute to equal 4 tablespoons sugar ☆
2 teaspoons coconut extract ☆
1 (4-serving) package JELL-O sugar-free vanilla cook & serve pudding mix
1 (4-serving) package JELL-O sugar-free cherry gelatin
2 cups (one 16-ounce can) tart red cherries, packed in water, drained and liquid reserved
1 cup (one 8-ounce can) crushed pineapple, packed in fruit juice, drained and liquid reserved
1¹/₂ cups Yoplait plain fat-free yogurt
¹/₃ cup Carnation Nonfat Dry Milk Powder
1¹/₂ cups Cool Whip Lite
3 tablespoons flaked coconut

Preheat oven to 415 degrees. Pat rolls into an ungreased 10-by-15-inch rimmed cookie sheet. Gently press dough to cover bottom of pan, being sure to seal perforations. Bake 6 to 8 minutes or until golden brown. Place cookie sheet on a wire rack and allow to cool. In a medium bowl, stir cream cheese with a spoon until soft. Stir in 2 tablespoons sugar substitute and 1 teaspoon coconut extract. Spread cream cheese mixture evenly over cooled crust. In a medium saucepan, combine dry pudding mix and dry gelatin. Add enough water to reserved cherry and pineapple liquids to make 1¼ cups liquid. Add liquid to pudding mixture. Mix well to combine. Stir in cherries and pineapple. Cook over medium heat, stirring constantly until mixture thickens and starts to boil. Remove from heat. Place pan on a wire rack and allow to cool completely. Spread cooled cherry mixture evenly over cream cheese mixture. In a medium bowl, combine yogurt and dry milk powder. Add remaining 1 teaspoon coconut extract and remaining 2 tablespoons sugar substitute. Blend in Cool Whip Lite. Spread topping mixture evenly over cherry filling. Evenly sprinkle coconut over top. Refrigerate at least 1 hour. Cut into 12 servings. Refrigerate any leftovers.

HINT:
Do not use inexpensive rolls. They don't cover the pan properly.

Each serving equals:

DIABETIC: 1 Starch • 1 Fat • ½ Fruit

156 Calories • 5 gm Fat • 6 gm Protein • 22 gm Carbohydrate • 358 mg Sodium • 1 gm Fiber

HE: ⅔ Bread • ½ Fruit • ⅓ Protein • ⅓ Skim Milk • ¼ Slider • 13 Optional Calories

Cherry Dessert Pizza

Pizza never tasted like this in the old days! Welcome to the future — and all that healthy desserts can be.

✌ Serves 8

> 1 refrigerated unbaked 9-inch Pillsbury piecrust
> 1 (4-serving) package JELL-O sugar-free vanilla cook & serve pudding mix
> 1 (4-serving) package JELL-O sugar-free cherry gelatin
> 1¹/₂ cups water
> 4 cups (two 16-ounce cans) tart red cherries, packed in water, drained
> 1 (8-ounce) package Philadelphia Fat Free Cream Cheese
> Sugar substitute to equal 2 tablespoons sugar
> 2 tablespoons (¹/₂ ounce) chopped pecans
> 1 teaspoon vanilla extract
> 1 cup Cool Whip Lite

Preheat oven to 350 degrees. Let piecrust warm to room temperature. Gently pat into a 12-inch pizza pan. Prick crust with fork evenly over bottom. Bake 30 minutes or until lightly browned. Place pizza pan on a wire rack and allow to cool 10 minutes. In a medium saucepan, combine dry pudding mix, dry gelatin, water, and cherries. Cook over medium heat, stirring constantly, until mixture thickens and starts to boil. Remove from heat. Place saucepan on a wire rack and allow to cool. In a medium bowl, stir cream cheese with a spoon until soft. Add sugar substitute, pecans, and vanilla extract. Mix well to combine. Spread cream cheese mixture over cooled crust. Evenly spread cooled cherry mixture over cream cheese mixture. Garnish top with Cool Whip Lite. Refrigerate at least 1 hour. Cut into 8 servings.

Each serving equals:

DIABETIC: 1 Fat • 1 Meat • 1 Starch • 1 Fruit
229 Calories • 9 gm Fat • 7 gm Protein • 30 gm Carbohydrate • 411 mg Sodium • 2 gm Fiber
HE: 1 Protein • 1 Fruit • 1/2 Bread • 1/4 Fat • 1 Slider • 6 Optional Calories

Cupid's Chocolate Cups

❋

Cupid would approve of this "love nectar" in tart crusts. It'll hit the mark with all chocolate lovers . . . and I bet there'll be a kiss for the cook!

✌ Serves 6

> 1 (4-serving) package JELL-O sugar-free instant chocolate pudding mix
> $^2/_3$ cup Carnation Nonfat Dry Milk Powder
> $^3/_4$ cup Yoplait plain fat-free yogurt
> 1 cup water
> $^1/_2$ teaspoon almond extract
> 1 (6-single serve) package Keebler graham cracker crusts
> 6 tablespoons Cool Whip Lite
> 3 maraschino cherries, halved

In a medium bowl, combine dry pudding mix and dry milk powder. Add yogurt, water, and almond extract. Mix well using a wire whisk. Evenly spoon pudding mixture into crusts. Top each with 1 tablespoon Cool Whip Lite and $^1/_2$ maraschino cherry. Refrigerate at least 1 hour.

Each serving equals:

DIABETIC: 1 Starch • 1 Fat • $^1/_2$ Skim Milk

182 Calories • 6 gm Fat • 6 gm Protein • 26 gm Carbohydrate • 406 mg Sodium • 1 gm Fiber

HE: $^1/_2$ Bread • $^1/_2$ Skim Milk • $^3/_4$ Slider • 14 Optional Calories

Southern Belle Tarts ✳

If it's true what they say about how irresistible and sweet those Southern ladies can be, then these pleasing treats are perfectly named!

✌ Serves 6

> 1 (4-serving) package JELL-O sugar-free instant vanilla pudding mix
> ²/₃ cup Carnation Nonfat Dry Milk Powder
> 1¹/₃ cups water
> 6 tablespoons apricot spreadable fruit spread
> 3 tablespoons (³/₄ ounce) chopped pecans
> 1 (6-single serve) package Keebler graham cracker crusts
> 6 tablespoons Cool Whip Lite

In a large bowl, combine dry pudding mix and dry milk powder. Add water. Mix well using a wire whisk. Blend in apricot spreadable fruit and pecans. Spoon mixture evenly into crusts. Top each with 1 tablespoon Cool Whip Lite. Refrigerate at least 1 hour.

Each serving equals:

DIABETIC: 1 Fruit • 1 Starch • ¹/₂ Skim Milk • ¹/₂ Fat

224 Calories • 8 gm Fat • 4 gm Protein • 34 gm Carbohydrate • 399 mg Sodium • 2 gm Fiber

HE: 1 Fruit • ¹/₂ Fat • ¹/₂ Bread • ¹/₃ Skim Milk • ³/₄ Slider • 15 Optional Calories

Pineapple Cream Tarts

Put on a Hawaiian shirt and think "vacation!" while eating these sunny tropical treats.

✌ Serves 6

> *1 cup (one 8-ounce can) crushed pineapple, packed in fruit juice, undrained*
> *1 (4-serving) package JELL-O sugar-free vanilla cook & serve pudding mix*
> *1 (4-serving) package JELL-O sugar-free lemon gelatin*
> *¹/₂ cup water*
> *1 (8-ounce) package Philadelphia Fat Free Cream Cheese*
> *Sugar substitute to equal 2 tablespoons sugar*
> *¹/₂ teaspoon coconut extract*
> *1 (6-single serve) package Keebler graham cracker crusts*
> *6 tablespoons Cool Whip Lite*
> *1 maraschino cherry*

In a medium saucepan, combine undrained pineapple, dry pudding mix, dry gelatin, and water. Cook over medium heat, stirring constantly, until mixture thickens and starts to boil. Remove from heat. Place pan on a wire rack and allow to cool completely. In a medium bowl, stir cream cheese with a spoon until soft. Stir in sugar substitute and coconut extract. Add cooled pineapple mixture. Mix gently, but thoroughly. Evenly spoon mixture into crusts. Top each with 1 tablespoon Cool Whip Lite. Cut cherry in half and each half into 3 pieces. Garnish each tart with a cherry piece. Refrigerate at least 1 hour.

Each serving equals:

DIABETIC: 1 Starch • 1 Fat • ¹/₂ Fruit • ¹/₂ Meat
197 Calories • 5 gm Fat • 12 gm Protein • 26 gm Carbohydrate • 545 mg Sodium • 1 gm Fiber
HE: 1 Bread • ²/₃ Protein • ¹/₃ Fruit • 1 Slider • 4 Optional Calories

Fresh Strawberry-Rhubarb Pie   ✳

The dictionary defines strawberry as (1) a small, juicy, red, edible fruit (2) the low plant of the rose family it grows on. I define strawberry as the most wonderful food on earth! If you share my love of strawberries, I think you will enjoy this recipe I created to let that glorious fruit shine.

✌ Serves 8

> 1 refrigerated unbaked 9-inch Pillsbury piecrust
> 1 (4-serving) package JELL-O sugar-free strawberry gelatin
> 1 (4-serving) package JELL-O sugar-free vanilla cook & serve pudding mix
> ¹/₂ cup water
> 2 cups finely chopped rhubarb
> 2 cups chopped fresh strawberries
> 6 tablespoons Bisquick Reduced Fat Baking Mix
> 2 tablespoons Sugar Twin or Sprinkle Sweet
> 1 tablespoon + 1 teaspoon reduced-calorie margarine

Preheat oven to 400 degrees. Place piecrust in a 9-inch pie plate and flute edges. Set aside. In a medium saucepan, combine dry gelatin, dry pudding mix, and water. Stir in rhubarb. Cook over medium heat, stirring often, until rhubarb is tender, about 8 minutes. Remove from heat. Place strawberries in bottom of prepared piecrust. Spoon hot rhubarb mixture evenly over strawberries. In a medium bowl, combine baking mix and Sugar Twin. Add margarine. Mix well with a fork until mixture is crumbly. Sprinkle mixture evenly over top of pie. Bake 15 minutes. Lower heat to 350 degrees and continue baking 45 minutes. Place pie plate on a wire rack and allow to cool completely. Cut into 8 servings.

HINT:

Good served with Cool Whip Lite, but don't forget to count the few additional calories.

Each serving equals:

DIABETIC: 1 Starch • 1 Fat • ½ Fruit

193 Calories • 9 gm Fat • 6 gm Protein • 22 gm Carbohydrate • 305 mg Sodium • 3 gm Fiber

HE: ¾ Bread • ½ Vegetable • ¼ Fruit • ¼ Fat • ¾ Slider • 6 Optional Calories

Rhubarb-Raspberry Chiffon Pie

I've given that old-time favorite, rhubarb chiffon, a new twist by adding raspberries. Yum!

✌ Serves 8

1 refrigerated unbaked 9-inch Pillsbury piecrust
4 cups cut rhubarb
²/₃ cup water
2 (4-serving) packages JELL-O sugar-free raspberry gelatin
1¹/₂ cups frozen unsweetened raspberries
¹/₄ cup Sugar Twin or Sprinkle Sweet
1 cup Cool Whip Lite

Preheat oven to 450 degrees. Place piecrust in a 9-inch pie plate. Flute edges and prick bottom and sides with a fork. Bake 9 to 11 minutes or until lightly browned. Place pie plate on a wire rack and allow to cool completely. Meanwhile, in a medium saucepan, combine rhubarb and water. Cover and cook over medium heat until rhubarb is tender, about 10 minutes. Remove from heat. Add dry gelatin. Mix well to dissolve gelatin. Stir in frozen raspberries. Place pan on a wire rack and allow to cool completely. Fold in Sugar Twin and Cool Whip Lite. Mix gently to combine. Pour rhubarb mixture into cooled piecrust. Refrigerate at least 2 hours. Cut into 8 servings.

Each serving equals:

DIABETIC: 1 Starch • 1 Fat • ½ Fruit

168 Calories • 8 gm Fat • 3 gm Protein • 21 gm Carbohydrate • 198 mg Sodium • 2 gm Fiber

HE: 1 Vegetable • ½ Bread • ¼ Fruit • ¾ Slider • 15 Optional Calories

Apple Surprise Pie

I've stirred so many surprises in this scrumptious pie that it will take a treasure map to find them all. But everyone will have fun trying.

✌ Serves 8

1 (4-serving) package JELL-O sugar-free instant butterscotch pudding mix
²/₃ cup Carnation Nonfat Dry Milk Powder
1 cup unsweetened apple juice
¹/₄ cup (1 ounce) chopped pecans
1 cup (2 small) unpeeled diced Red Delicious apples
¹/₂ cup (1 ounce) miniature marshmallows
1 (6-ounce) Keebler chocolate-flavored piecrust
³/₄ cup Cool Whip Lite
1 tablespoon (¹/₄ ounce) mini chocolate chips

In a medium bowl, combine dry pudding mix and dry milk powder. Add apple juice. Mix well using a wire whisk. Blend in pecans, apples, and marshmallows. Spread mixture evenly into piecrust. Refrigerate 30 minutes. Evenly spread Cool Whip Lite over filling. Sprinkle chocolate chips evenly over top. Refrigerate at least 1 hour. Cut into 8 servings.

Each serving equals:

DIABETIC: 1 Starch • 1 Fruit • 1 Fat

211 Calories • 7 gm Fat • 3 gm Protein • 34 gm Carbohydrate • 298 mg Sodium • 2 gm Fiber

HE: ¹/₂ Bread • ¹/₂ Fruit • ¹/₄ Fat • ¹/₄ Skim Milk • 1 Slider • 8 Optional Calories

Caribbean Queen Cream Pie

It just doesn't get any better than a strawberry-and-banana duo. Add pineapple, and you have a winner in just about anyone's mouth. If you've never visited the islands, this will give you a taste of how sweet it can be!

✌ Serves 8

1 cup (1 medium) sliced banana
1 cup sliced fresh strawberries
1 (6-ounce) Keebler graham cracker piecrust
1 (4-serving) package JELL-O sugar-free instant banana pudding mix
²/₃ cup Carnation Nonfat Dry Milk Powder
1 cup (one 8-ounce can) crushed pineapple, packed in fruit juice, drained and liquid reserved
³/₄ cup Cool Whip Lite ☆
¹/₂ teaspoon rum extract
1 teaspoon coconut extract
2 tablespoons flaked coconut

Layer bananas and strawberries in bottom of piecrust. In a medium bowl, combine dry pudding mix and dry milk powder. Add enough water to reserved pineapple juice to make 1¹/₃ cups liquid. Add liquid to dry pudding mixture. Mix well using a wire whisk. Blend in ¹/₄ cup Cool Whip Lite and rum extract. Spread pudding mixture evenly over fruit. Refrigerate while preparing topping. In a small bowl, combine pineapple, remaining ½ cup Cool Whip Lite, and coconut extract. Mix gently to combine. Frost top of pie with pineapple mixture. Evenly sprinkle coconut over the top. Refrigerate at least 1 hour. Cut into 8 servings.

Each serving equals:

DIABETIC: 1 Starch • 1 Fruit • 1 Fat

207 Calories • 7 gm Fat • 3 gm Protein • 34 gm Carbohydrate • 349 mg Sodium • 2 gm Fiber

HE: ½ Bread • ½ Fruit • ¼ Skim Milk • 1 Slider • 2 Optional Calories

Peach Becky Pie

A wonderful pie named in honor of a wonderful daughter. Becky's favorite fruit is fresh peaches. She's pleased with her namesake and is glad to share the flavors in this pie with you.

❦ Serves 8

> 1 (4-serving) package JELL-O sugar-free instant vanilla pudding mix
> ⅔ cup Carnation Nonfat Dry Milk Powder
> 1¼ cups water
> 1 cup Cool Whip Lite ☆
> 2 cups peeled and chopped fresh peaches
> 1 (6-ounce) Keebler butter-flavored piecrust
> ¼ cup raspberry spreadable fruit spread

In a large bowl, combine dry pudding mix and dry milk powder. Add water. Mix well using a wire whisk. Blend in ½ cup Cool Whip Lite. Add chopped peaches. Mix gently to combine. Spread mixture evenly into piecrust. Refrigerate while preparing topping. In a small bowl, stir raspberry spreadable fruit until soft. Add remaining ½ cup Cool Whip Lite. Mix gently to combine. Spread topping mixture evenly over set filling. Refrigerate at least 2 hours. Cut into 8 servings.

Each serving equals:

DIABETIC: 1 Starch • 1 Fruit • 1 Fat

194 Calories • 6 gm Fat • 3 gm Protein • 32 gm Carbohydrate • 323 mg Sodium • 2 gm Fiber

HE: ³/₄ Fruit • ¹/₂ Bread • ¹/₄ Skim Milk • 1 Slider • 3 Optional Calories

Irish Spring Pie

Here's a dessert as fresh and radiant as a spring morn in Ireland. County Mayo, to be exact. (That's where my family hails from.) *Erin go bragh!*

✌ Serves 8

1 (8-ounce) package Philadelphia Fat Free Cream Cheese
1 cup (one 8-ounce can) crushed pineapple, packed in fruit juice, well drained
Sugar substitute to equal 2 tablespoons sugar
1/2 teaspoon coconut extract
1 (6-ounce) Keebler butter-flavored piecrust
2 cups (2 medium) sliced bananas
1 (4-serving) package JELL-O sugar-free instant pistachio pudding mix
2/3 cup Carnation Nonfat Dry Milk Powder
1 1/3 cups water
1/2 cup Cool Whip Lite
2 tablespoons flaked coconut

In a large bowl, stir cream cheese with a spoon until soft. Add pineapple, sugar substitute, and coconut extract. Mix gently to combine. Spread mixture evenly in bottom of piecrust. Layer sliced bananas over cream cheese mixture. In a medium bowl, combine dry pudding mix and dry milk powder. Add water. Mix well using a wire whisk. Blend in Cool Whip Lite. Pour pudding mixture evenly over bananas. Sprinkle coconut evenly over top. Refrigerate at least 2 hours. Cut into 8 servings.

Each serving equals:

DIABETIC: 1 Fruit • 1 Fat • 1 Starch • ¹/₂ Meat • ¹/₂ Skim Milk

272 Calories • 8 gm Fat • 10 gm Protein • 40 gm Carbohydrate • 546 mg Sodium • 2 gm Fiber

HE: ³/₄ Fruit • ¹/₂ Bread • ¹/₂ Protein • ¹/₄ Skim Milk • ³/₄ Slider • 18 Optional Calories

Pistachio Pizazz Pie ✳

This elegant, colorful pie is so easy that you'll want to make it often. The combination of pineapple with pistachio pudding is one my family asks for often — and I bet yours will, too.

✌ Serves 8

   2 cups (2 medium) sliced bananas
   1 (6-ounce) Keebler butter-flavored piecrust
   1 (4-serving) package JELL-O sugar-free instant
      pistachio pudding mix
   ²/₃ cup Carnation Nonfat Dry Milk Powder
   1 cup (one 8-ounce can) crushed pineapple, packed
      in fruit juice, undrained
   1 cup water
   1 cup Cool Whip Lite ☆

Layer bananas in bottom of piecrust. In a medium bowl, combine dry pudding mix and dry milk powder. Add undrained pineapple and water. Mix well using a wire whisk. Blend in ¹/₂ cup Cool Whip Lite. Pour pudding mixture evenly over bananas. Refrigerate at least 1 hour. Cut into 8 servings. When serving, top each piece with 1 tablespoon Cool Whip Lite.

Each serving equals:

DIABETIC: 1 Starch • 1 Fruit • 1 Fat

219 Calories • 7 gm Fat • 3 gm Protein • 36 gm Carbohydrate • 322 mg Sodium • 2 gm Fiber

HE: ³/₄ Fruit • ¹/₂ Bread • ¹/₄ Skim Milk • 1 Slider • 2 Optional Calories

Mint Patty Pie ✳

This tastes almost like a mint patty candy . . . only better!

✌ Serves 8

  1 (4-serving) package JELL-O sugar-free instant
    chocolate pudding mix
  $2/3$ cup Carnation Nonfat Dry Milk Powder
  $1^1/3$ cups water
  1 cup Cool Whip Lite ☆
  1 (6-ounce) Keebler chocolate-flavored piecrust
  $3/4$ teaspoon mint extract
  3 to 4 drops green food coloring
  1 tablespoon ($^1/4$ ounce) mini chocolate chips

In a medium bowl, combine dry pudding mix and dry milk powder. Add water. Mix well using a wire whisk. Blend in $1/4$ cup Cool Whip Lite. Pour mixture into piecrust. Refrigerate while preparing topping. In a small bowl, combine remaining $3/4$ cup Cool Whip Lite, mint extract, and green food coloring. Spread topping mixture evenly over set filling. Sprinkle chocolate chips evenly over top. Refrigerate at least 1 hour. Cut into 8 servings.

Each serving equals:

DIABETIC: $1^1/2$ Starch • 1 Fat

192 Calories • 8 gm Fat • 4 gm Protein • 26 gm Carbohydrate • 341 mg Sodium • 1 gm Fiber

HE: $1/2$ Bread • $1/4$ Skim Milk • 1 Slider • 10 Optional Calories

Chocolate "Ice Cream" Sundae Pie ✳

This frozen sensation tastes and looks so good, it's really quite an impressive dessert. The kid in all of us never really gets tired of the flavors in a chocolate sundae.

✌ Serves 8

1 (4-serving) package JELL-O sugar-free instant chocolate pudding mix
⅓ cup Carnation Nonfat Dry Milk Powder
1 cup skim milk
1 cup Cool Whip Lite ☆
1 teaspoon vanilla extract
1 (6-ounce) Keebler chocolate-flavored piecrust
2 teaspoons chocolate syrup
4 maraschino cherries, halved

In a large bowl, combine dry pudding mix and dry milk powder. Add skim milk. Mix well using a wire whisk. Blend in ½ cup Cool Whip Lite and vanilla extract. Pour mixture into piecrust. Refrigerate 10 minutes. Spread remaining ½ cup Cool Whip Lite evenly over set filling. Drizzle chocolate syrup over top and garnish with cherry halves. Cover and freeze. Remove from freezer about 15 minutes before serving. Cut into 8 servings.

Each serving equals:

DIABETIC: 1½ Starch • 1 Fat

187 Calories • 7 gm Fat • 4 gm Protein • 27 gm Carbohydrate • 293 mg Sodium • 1 gm Fiber

HE: ½ Bread • ¼ Skim Milk • 1 Slider • 12 Optional Calories

Heavenly Hash Pie ✳

Who would have ever thought that plain yogurt could turn into something so heavenly? You'll find that the pleasures in this pie bring out the angel in your kids — at least until dessert is served!

✌ Serves 8

> 1 (4-serving) package JELL-O sugar-free instant banana pudding mix
> $^1/_3$ cup Carnation Nonfat Dry Milk Powder
> $^3/_4$ cup Yoplait plain fat-free yogurt
> $^3/_4$ cup water
> $^1/_2$ teaspoon coconut extract
> 1 cup Cool Whip Lite ☆
> 1 cup (one 11-ounce can) mandarin oranges, rinsed and drained
> 1 cup (one 8-ounce can) pineapple chunks, packed in fruit juice, drained
> 1 (6-ounce) Keebler butter-flavored piecrust
> 1 tablespoon flaked coconut

In a large bowl, combine dry pudding mix and dry milk powder. Add yogurt and water. Mix well using a wire whisk. Stir in coconut extract, $^1/_4$ cup Cool Whip Lite, mandarin oranges, and pineapple. Pour mixture into piecrust. Refrigerate about 2 hours. Spread remaining $^3/_4$ cup Cool Whip Lite evenly over set filling. Sprinkle flaked coconut over top. Cut into 8 servings.

Each serving equals:

DIABETIC: 1 Starch • 1 Fruit • 1 Fat

201 Calories • 6 gm Fat • 4 gm Protein • 33 gm Carbohydrate • 336 mg Sodium • 1 gm Fiber

HE: ½ Bread • ½ Fruit • ¼ Skim Milk • 1 Slider • 4 Optional Calories

Scrumptious Surprise Lemon Pie ❋

If lemon is on your most preferred list of flavors, then this is the pie for you. Lemon lovers everywhere have endorsed this truly luscious pie.

✌ Serves 8

> 1 (8-ounce) package Philadelphia Fat Free Cream Cheese
> Sugar substitute to equal 2 tablespoons sugar
> 1 teaspoon vanilla extract
> 1 cup Cool Whip Lite ☆
> 1 (6-ounce) Keebler butter-flavored piecrust
> ¹/₄ cup (1 ounce) chopped pecans
> 1 (4-serving) package JELL-O sugar-free instant vanilla pudding mix
> 1 (4-serving) package JELL-O sugar-free lemon gelatin
> ²/₃ cup Carnation Nonfat Dry Milk Powder ☆
> 1¹/₃ cups water

In a large bowl, stir cream cheese with a spoon until soft. Add sugar substitute, vanilla extract, and ¹/₄ cup Cool Whip Lite. Mix well to combine. Spread mixture evenly into piecrust. Evenly sprinkle pecans over cream cheese mixture. In a medium bowl, combine dry pudding mix, dry gelatin, dry milk powder, and water. Mix well using a wire whisk. Spread pudding mixture evenly over pecans. Evenly spread remaining ³/₄ cup Cool Whip Lite over top. Refrigerate at least

2 hours. Cut into 8 servings.

Each serving equals:

DIABETIC: 1¹/₂ Starch • 1 Fat • ¹/₂ Meat
208 Calories • 8 gm Fat • 8 gm Protein • 26 gm
Carbohydrate • 424 mg Sodium • 1 gm Fiber
HE: ¹/₂ Bread • ¹/₂ Fat • ¹/₂ Protein • ¹/₄ Skim Milk
• 1 Slider • 9 Optional Calories

Washington's Cherry Cheesecake ✳

I think George would enjoy attending a party in his honor where this cheesecake was served, even though its low-fat/low-sugar ingredients were not even imagined during his lifetime. Let's hear it for good old American ingenuity! We've come a long way in a short time.

✌ Serves 8

> 2 (8-ounce) packages Philadelphia Fat Free Cream Cheese
> 1 (4-serving) package JELL-O sugar-free instant vanilla pudding mix
> ¾ cup Yoplait plain fat-free yogurt
> 1 cup skim milk
> 1½ teaspoons coconut extract ☆
> 1 (6-ounce) Keebler graham cracker piecrust
> 2 cups (one 16-ounce can) tart red cherries, packed in water, drained
> 1 (4-serving) package JELL-O sugar-free vanilla cook & serve pudding mix
> 1 (4-serving) package JELL-O sugar-free cherry gelatin
> 1¼ cups water

In a medium bowl, stir cream cheese with a spoon until soft. Add dry instant pudding mix, yogurt, skim milk, and 1 teaspoon coconut extract. Mix well using a wire whisk. Spread mixture evenly into piecrust. Cover and refrigerate. Meanwhile, in a medium saucepan, combine cherries, dry cook-and-serve pudding mix, dry gelatin, and water. Cook over medium heat, stirring constantly, until mixture thickens and starts to boil. Remove from heat. Stir in remaining 1/2 teaspoon coconut extract. Place pan on a wire rack and allow to cool completely. When ready to serve, cut cheesecake into 8 servings. Top each serving with about 1/4 cup of cherry sauce.

HINT:

Good topped with 1 tablespoon Cool Whip Lite. If using, don't forget to count the few additional calories.

Each serving equals:

DIABETIC: 1½ Starch • 1 Meat • ½ Fat • ½ Fruit

238 Calories • 5 gm Fat • 16 gm Protein • 32 gm Carbohydrate • 716 mg Sodium • 1 gm Fiber

HE: 1 Protein • ½ Bread • ¼ Skim Milk • ¼ Fruit • ¾ Slider • 19 Optional Calories

Pumpkin Cheesecake with
Cranberry Glaze ✳

I wanted to take the foods the Pilgrims would have eaten but prepare them in ways as modern as the twenty-first century. This cheesecake is the result. Lucky you — you don't have to cross an ocean to enjoy this updated pumpkin and cranberry treat.

❧ Serves 12

> 12 (2½-inch square) graham crackers
> 2 (8-ounce) packages Philadelphia Fat Free
>   Cream Cheese
> 1 (4-serving) package JELL-O sugar-free instant
>   vanilla pudding mix
> 2 cups (one 16-ounce can) pumpkin
> 1 teaspoon pumpkin pie spice
> 1¼ cups Cool Whip Lite ☆
> 1 (4-serving) package JELL-O sugar-free vanilla
>   cook & serve pudding mix
> 1 cup Ocean Spray Reduced Calorie Cranberry
>   Juice Cocktail
> ½ cup water
> 3 cups fresh cranberries

Evenly arrange graham crackers in a 9-by-13-inch cake pan. In a large bowl, stir cream cheese with a spoon until soft. Add dry instant pudding mix, pumpkin, and pumpkin pie spice. Mix well using a wire whisk. Fold in ½ cup Cool Whip Lite.

Carefully spread pumpkin mixture over graham crackers. Refrigerate. Meanwhile, in a medium saucepan, combine dry cook-and-serve pudding mix, cranberry juice cocktail, water, and cranberries. Cook over medium heat, stirring constantly, until mixture thickens and cranberries become soft. Place saucepan on a wire rack and allow to cool 20 minutes. Evenly spoon cooled cranberry mixture over pumpkin layer. Refrigerate at least 2 hours. Cut into 12 servings. When serving, top each piece with 1 tablespoon Cool Whip Lite.

Each serving equals:

DIABETIC: 1 Starch • ½ Meat

109 Calories • 1 gm Fat • 6 gm Protein • 19 gm Carbohydrate • 428 mg Sodium • 2 gm Fiber

HE: ⅔ Protein • ½ Bread • ⅓ Vegetable • ⅓ Fruit • ¼ Slider • 12 Optional Calories

Pistachio Cheesecake with Pineapple-Strawberry Glaze

Until you've tried this pistachio cheesecake, you haven't tried the best! The combination of flavors and colors is truly something special to behold.

✌ Serves 8

> 9 (2¹/₂-inch square) graham crackers
> 2 (8-ounce) packages Philadelphia Fat Free Cream Cheese
> 2 cups skim milk ☆
> 2 (4-serving) packages JELL-O sugar-free instant pistachio pudding mix
> 1 cup (one 8-ounce can) crushed pineapple, packed in fruit juice, undrained
> ³/₄ cup water
> 1 (4-serving) package JELL-O sugar-free strawberry gelatin
> 1 tablespoon + 1 teaspoon cornstarch
> 2 cups sliced fresh strawberries

Evenly arrange graham crackers in a 9-by-9-inch cake pan. In a large bowl, stir cream cheese with a spoon until soft. Blend in ¹/₂ cup skim milk. Add remaining 1¹/₂ cups skim milk and dry pudding mixes. Mix well using a wire whisk. Spread cream cheese mixture evenly over graham crackers. Refrigerate. Meanwhile, in a medium saucepan, combine undrained pineapple and water. Add dry gelatin and cornstarch. Cook over medium heat, stirring constantly, until mixture thickens and starts to boil. Remove from heat. Gently stir in strawberries. Place saucepan on a wire rack and allow to cool 20 minutes. Evenly spread cooled strawberry mixture over pudding mixture. Refrigerate at least 1 hour. Cut into 8 servings.

Each serving equals:

DIABETIC: 1 Meat • 1 Starch • ½ Fruit

154 Calories • 2 gm Fat • 11 gm Protein • 23 gm Carbohydrate • 458 mg Sodium • 1 gm Fiber

HE: 1 Protein • ½ Fruit • ⅓ Bread • ¼ Skim Milk • ¼ Slider • 15 Optional Calories

This 'n' That

Cucumber Canapés

I don't think I have ever been to a party that didn't have some type of finger sandwich on the buffet. These may be just what you have been looking for to serve at your next party.

✌ Serves 16 (3 each)

> 1 (8-ounce) package Philadelphia Fat Free Cream Cheese
> 2 tablespoons Kraft fat-free mayonnaise
> 1 to 2 drops Tabasco sauce
> 2 teaspoons Italian seasoning
> 48 pumpernickel bread rounds or squares
> 48 unpeeled cucumber slices
> Paprika

In a medium bowl, stir cream cheese with a spoon until soft. Add mayonnaise, Tabasco sauce, and Italian seasoning. Mix well to combine. Spread about 1 full teaspoon mixture on each bread round. Place cucumber slice on each. Lightly sprinkle tops with paprika. Cover and refrigerate at least 1 hour.

Each serving equals:

DIABETIC: 1 Starch

93 Calories • 1 gm Fat • 5 gm Protein • 16 gm Carbohydrate • 293 mg Sodium • 1 gm Fiber

HE: 1 Bread • 1/4 Protein • 1/4 Vegetable

Shrimp-Stuffed Celery

Here's another delicious finger food for your guests to munch on. You don't have to tell them it's healthy. They won't suspect a thing.

✌ Serves 8 (8 pieces each)

1 (8-ounce) package *Philadelphia Fat Free Cream Cheese*
¼ cup Kraft fat-free mayonnaise
2 tablespoons Kraft Fat Free French Dressing
1 (4.5 ounce drained weight) can small shrimp, rinsed, drained, and chopped
1 teaspoon dried parsley flakes
16 (4-inch) pieces crisp celery

In a medium bowl, stir cream cheese with a spoon until soft. Add mayonnaise and French dressing. Mix well to combine. Stir in shrimp and parsley flakes. Pack grooves of celery with mixture. Cut each celery strip crosswise into 1-inch pieces. Cover and refrigerate at least 1 hour.

Each serving equals:

DIABETIC: 1 Vegetable • 1 Meat

48 Calories • 0 gm Fat • 7 gm Protein • 5 gm Carbohydrate • 321 mg Sodium • 0 gm Fiber

HE: 1 Vegetable • 1 Protein • 8 Optional Calories

Cherry Pie Filling

I've had so many requests for my recipe for sugar-free cherry pie filling that's almost as fast as opening up a store-bought can. Now, start imagining with me . . . if you can prepare cherry pie filling this easily, doesn't it stand to reason that you could stir up the fruit filling of your choice by using an appropriate flavor gelatin and your choice of canned fruits? Yes, you can!

Serves 8

1 (4-serving) package JELL-O sugar-free vanilla cook & serve pudding mix
1 (4-serving) package JELL-O sugar-free cherry gelatin
1¼ cups water
2 cups (one 16-ounce can) tart red cherries, packed in water, drained

In a medium saucepan, combine dry pudding mix, dry gelatin, water, and cherries. Cook over medium heat, stirring constantly, until mixture thickens and starts to boil. Remove from heat. Place pan on a wire rack and allow to cool completely. Use as you would purchased canned cherry pie filling.

HINT:
After removing mixture from heat, try adding ½ teaspoon almond extract. It's wonderful!

Each serving equals:

DIABETIC: ½ Fruit

45 Calories • less than 1 gm Fat • 4 gm Protein • 7 gm Carbohydrate • 102 mg Sodium • 1 gm Fiber

HE: ½ Fruit • 14 Optional Calories

Banana-Strawberry Topping

As a card-carrying member of the I Love Strawberries Club, I highly recommend this marvelous strawberry sauce. This is great as is or served over fat-free ice cream, shortcake, and even on top of pancakes or french toast.

✌ Serves 4 (½ cup)

2 cups sliced fresh strawberries ☆
¼ cup Sugar Twin or Sprinkle Sweet
1 cup (1 medium) diced banana

In a medium bowl, mash ½ cup strawberries using a fork or potato masher. Blend in Sugar Twin. Add banana and remaining strawberries. Mix well to combine. Cover and refrigerate. Gently stir again just before serving.

Each serving equals:

DIABETIC: 1 Fruit

54 Calories • 0 gm Fat • 1 gm Protein • 13 gm Carbohydrate • 4 mg Sodium • 3 gm Fiber

HE: 1 Fruit • 6 Optional Calories

Adobe Hacienda Egg Bake

This easy egg dish was an early-morning winner with Cliff, who has high standards when it comes to breakfast. He even wanted it again the next day. But no such luck, I had to tell him. I was already on to other creations.

❧ Serves 8

> 6 eggs, beaten, or equivalent in egg substitute
> ³/₄ cup chunky salsa ☆
> 1 teaspoon dried parsley flakes
> ¹/₂ cup Kraft fat-free mayonnaise
> ¹/₄ cup chopped green bell pepper
> Scant 1 cup (2 ounces) corn chips, slightly crushed
> ¹/₂ cup Land O Lakes no-fat sour cream

Preheat oven to 350 degrees. Spray a 9-inch pie plate with olive-flavored cooking spray. In a large bowl, combine eggs, ¹/₄ cup salsa, parsley flakes, and mayonnaise. Add green pepper and corn chips. Mix gently to combine. Pour mixture into prepared pie plate. Bake 25 to 30 minutes or until knife inserted in center comes out clean. Place pie plate on a wire rack and let set 5 minutes. Cut into 8 servings. For each serving, place 1 piece on plate and top with 1 tablespoon salsa and 1 tablespoon sour cream.

Each serving equals:

DIABETIC: 1 Meat • ½ Starch • ½ Fat

123 Calories • 6 gm Fat • 6 gm Protein • 11 gm Carbohydrate • 325 mg Sodium • 0 gm Fiber

HE: ¾ Protein (limited) • ¼ Vegetable • ¼ Bread • ½ Slider • 3 Optional Calories

Ham-and-Apple-Topped Biscuits ✳

What a special way to start the day! But remember that this sweet and tangy dish is just as good at lunch or supper.

✌ Serves 4

> 1 full cup (6 ounces) diced Dubuque 97% fat-free ham or any extra-lean ham
> 1 cup (2 small) unpeeled chopped cooking apples
> 1/4 cup raisins
> 2/3 cup Cary's Sugar Free Maple Syrup
> 1/2 teaspoon apple pie spice
> 4 warm baked Pillsbury refrigerated buttermilk biscuits

In a large skillet sprayed with butter-flavored cooking spray, sauté ham and apples over medium heat for 5 minutes, stirring occasionally. Add raisins, maple syrup, and apple pie spice. Mix well to combine. Lower heat and simmer 2 to 3 minutes. For each serving, place 1 biscuit on plate and spoon about 1/2 cup ham mixture over top.

HINT:
> Bake entire package of biscuits. Freeze unused cooled biscuits for future use. They warm up great in the microwave.

Each serving equals:

DIABETIC: 1 Fruit • 1 Meat • 1 Starch

215 Calories • 6 gm Fat • 10 gm Protein • 30 gm Carbohydrate • 694 mg Sodium • 2 gm Fiber

HE: 1 Fruit • 1 Protein • 1 Bread • $^1/_4$ Slider • 7 Optional Calories

Pecan Pancakes with Pineapple Topping ✳

A delightful treat for any meal — elegant enough to serve to company but easy enough to prepare just for your family. Everyone will make time for breakfast when these appear on the table.

✌ Serves 4

> 1 cup (one 8-ounce can) crushed pineapple, packed
>   in fruit juice, undrained
> $^1/_4$ cup apple butter
> 1 cup Aunt Jemima Reduced Calorie Pancake Mix
> $^3/_4$ cup water
> 2 tablespoons ($^1/_2$ ounce) chopped pecans

In a medium saucepan, combine undrained pineapple and apple butter. Cook over low heat, stirring occasionally. Meanwhile, in a medium bowl, combine pancake mix, water, and pecans. Using a $^1/_3$-cup measure as a guide, pour batter on large hot skillet or griddle sprayed with butter-flavored cooking spray, to form 4 pancakes. Brown pancakes on both sides. For each serving, place a pancake on plate, quickly spray top with butter-flavored cooking spray, and spoon about $^1/_4$ cup warm pineapple mixture over top.

Each serving equals:

DIABETIC: 1½ Starch • 1 Fruit • ½ Fat

200 Calories • 4 gm Fat • 0 gm Protein • 39 gm Carbohydrate • 331 mg Sodium • 4 gm Fiber

HE: 1¾ Bread • ½ Fat • ¼ Fruit • 15 Optional Calories

Creamy Thousand Island Dip

This concoction is creamy, colorful, and perfect for dunking veggies and fat-free crackers.

✌ Serves 8 (¹/₄ cup)

> ³/₄ cup Yoplait plain fat-free yogurt
> ¹/₃ cup Carnation Nonfat Dry Milk Powder
> ¹/₄ cup Kraft fat-free mayonnaise
> 3 tablespoons chili sauce
> 2 tablespoons chopped green bell pepper
> 2 tablespoons chopped pimiento
> 2 tablespoons sweet pickle relish

In a medium bowl, combine yogurt and dry milk powder. Add mayonnaise. Mix well to combine. Stir in chili sauce, green pepper, pimiento, and pickle relish. Cover and refrigerate. Gently stir again just before serving.

Each serving equals:

DIABETIC: ¹/₂ Skim Milk *or* ¹/₂ Starch

40 Calories • 0 gm Fat • 2 gm Protein • 8 gm Carbohydrate • 207 mg Sodium • 0 gm Fiber

HE: ¹/₄ Skim Milk • 15 Optional Calories

Caramel Apple Dip

Serve this with sliced apples. It's almost as good, if not better, than a taffy apple (and with much less guilt).

✌ Serves 8 (¹/₄ cup)

1 (4-serving) package JELL-O sugar-free vanilla cook & serve pudding mix
1 (4-serving) package JELL-O sugar-free lemon gelatin
¹/₄ cup Brown Sugar Twin
1 teaspoon apple pie spice
1¹/₄ cups water
1 teaspoon vanilla extract
1 (8-ounce) package Philadelphia Fat Free Cream Cheese
¹/₄ cup (1 ounce) finely chopped dry-roasted peanuts

In a medium saucepan, combine dry pudding mix, dry gelatin, Brown Sugar Twin, apple pie spice, and water. Cook over medium heat, stirring constantly, until mixture thickens and starts to boil. Remove from heat. Stir in vanilla extract. Place pan on a wire rack and allow to cool 5 minutes. Meanwhile, in a medium bowl, stir cream cheese with a spoon until soft. Add chopped peanuts. Mix well to combine. Stir in slightly cooled pudding mixture. Refrigerate at least 1 hour. Gently stir again just before serving.

Each serving equals:

DIABETIC: 1 Meat

62 Calories • 2 gm Fat • 6 gm Protein • 5 gm Carbohydrate • 271 mg Sodium • 0 gm Fiber

HE: $^2/_3$ Protein • $^1/_4$ Fat • 17 Optional Calories

Fluffy Fruit Dip

This dip is so good with fresh fruit. Try it with sliced strawberries, pineapple, and peaches, for a party or just an easy dinner with friends.

✌ Serves 8 (¼ cup)

> 1 (4-serving) package JELL-O sugar-free vanilla cook & serve pudding mix
> 1 (4-serving) package JELL-O sugar-free mixed fruit gelatin
> 1¼ cups water
> 1 (8-ounce) package Philadelphia Fat Free Cream Cheese

In a medium saucepan, combine dry pudding mix, dry gelatin, and water. Cook over medium heat, stirring constantly, until mixture thickens and starts to boil. Remove from heat. Place pan on a wire rack and allow to cool 5 minutes. Stir in cream cheese. Mix well to combine. Refrigerate. Just before serving, let set at room temperature 10 minutes, then gently stir.

Each serving equals:

DIABETIC: ½ Meat

39 Calories • 0 gm Fat • 5 gm Protein • 4 gm Carbohydrate • 267 mg Sodium • 0 gm Fiber

HE: ½ Protein • 14 Optional Calories

Little Grass Hut Colada

You just may jump up and do the hula after sipping this refreshing drink!

✌ Serves 4 (1 cup)

> *1 cup (1 medium) sliced banana*
> *1 cup (one 8-ounce can) crushed pineapple, packed in fruit juice, undrained*
> *Sugar substitute to equal 2 tablespoons sugar*
> *1 teaspoon coconut extract*
> *2 cups cold Diet 7UP ☆*
> *1 cup chopped ice*

In a blender container, combine banana, pineapple, sugar substitute, coconut extract, 1 cup Diet 7UP, and chopped ice. Cover and process on HIGH 20 to 30 seconds or until mixture is smooth. Stir in remaining 1 cup Diet 7UP. Serve at once.

Each serving equals:

DIABETIC: 1 Fruit

72 Calories • 0 gm Fat • less than 1 gm Protein • 17 gm Carbohydrate • 18 mg Sodium • 1 gm Fiber

HE: 1 Fruit • 4 Optional Calories

Lemon-Strawberry Punch

Be prepared to share the recipe for this easy punch whenever you serve it! The fresh strawberries give it a special flavor.

✌ Serves 12 (1 full cup)

3 cups sliced fresh strawberries
1 tub Crystal Light sugar-free lemonade mix
8 cups very cold water ☆
Sugar substitute to equal 1/4 cup sugar
4 cups cold Diet 7UP

In a blender container, process strawberries on PUREE 20 seconds. Add dry lemonade mix, 2 cups water, and sugar substitute. Cover and process on BLEND 15 seconds or until mixture is smooth. Pour mixture into punch bowl. Add remaining 6 cups water and Diet 7UP. Mix well to combine. Serve at once or store in refrigerator until ready to serve.

Each serving equals:

DIABETIC: 1 Free Food

13 Calories • 0 gm Fat • 0 gm Protein • 3 gm Carbohydrate • 13 mg Sodium • 0 gm Fiber

HE: 1/4 Fruit • 8 Optional Calories

Goblin's Apple Brew

Stir up a batch of this and watch the smiles appear. The perfect after-school or after-work snack in a glass!

✌ Serves 4 (1 cup)

> 2 cups unsweetened apple juice
> 1½ cups Diet Mountain Dew
> 1 (4-serving) package JELL-O sugar-free instant vanilla pudding mix
> ½ teaspoon apple pie spice
> ¼ cup Cool Whip Lite
> ½ cup chopped ice

In a blender container, combine apple juice and Diet Mountain Dew. Add dry pudding mix and apple pie spice. Cover and process on BLEND 15 seconds. Add Cool Whip Lite and continue to process on BLEND another 15 seconds. Gradually add ice and process on HIGH until smooth, about 15 seconds. Serve at once.

Each serving equals:

DIABETIC: 1½ Fruit

87 Calories • less than 1 gm Fat • 0 gm Protein • 21 gm Carbohydrate • 337 mg Sodium • 0 gm Fiber

HE: 1 Fruit • ¼ Slider • 12 Optional Calories

Eggnog

Eggnog MUST be served at all holiday functions. Isn't that the law of the land? Well, here's my version — prepared without eggs, sugar, fat, or liquor, it still tastes exactly like traditional eggnog.

✌ Serves 4 (1 cup)

  4 cups skim milk
  *1 (4-serving) package JELL-O sugar-free instant
    vanilla pudding mix*
  ¹/₂ teaspoon rum extract
  ¹/₄ teaspoon ground nutmeg

In a large pitcher, combine skim milk, dry pudding mix, rum extract, and nutmeg. Mix well using a long spoon. Refrigerate 5 minutes. Gently stir again. Serve at once.

HINT:
  If you like thinner eggnog, add 1 cup of cold water when adding skim milk.

Each serving equals:

DIABETIC: 1 Skim Milk • ¹/₂ Starch
104 Calories • 0 gm Fat • 8 gm Protein • 18 gm Carbohydrate • 446 mg Sodium • 0 gm Fiber
HE: 1 Skim Milk • ¹/₄ Slider • 5 Optional Calories

Hot Spiced Cider

It tastes just like hot apple pie in a cup, but without the apples! Try it and see.

✌ Serves 8 (full ½ cup)

4 cups unsweetened apple juice
¹/₄ cup Brown Sugar Twin
1 cup water
1 teaspoon apple pie spice

In a medium saucepan, combine apple juice, Brown Sugar Twin, and water. Bring mixture to a boil. Stir in apple pie spice. Lower heat and simmer 30 minutes.

Each serving equals:

DIABETIC: 1 Fruit

60 Calories • 0 gm Fat • 0 gm Protein • 15 gm Carbohydrate • 7 mg Sodium • 0 gm Fiber

HE: 1 Fruit • 3 Optional Calories

Happy Trails Popcorn Mix

You don't have to roam the range to munch on this tasty snack. Just kick back watching a Western movie with some of this mix and see if you don't lasso a few "yippie-iy-ky-yays"!

✌ Serves 12 (1 cup)

9 cups air-popped popcorn
I Can't Believe It's Not Butter spray
1 cup raisins
1¹/₃ cups (6 ounces) chopped dried apricots
¹/₂ cup (2 ounces) chopped pecans
1 cup (2 ounces) mini marshmallows
1 teaspoon ground cinnamon
2 tablespoons Brown Sugar Twin

Place popped popcorn in a large bowl and quickly spray with I Can't Believe It's Not Butter spray. Stir in raisins, apricots, pecans, and marshmallows. Sprinkle cinnamon and Brown Sugar Twin over top. Mix well to combine. Store in airtight container.

HINTS:
1. To plump up raisins without "cooking," place in a glass measuring cup and microwave on HIGH for 30 seconds.
2. Six tablespoons unpopped popcorn usually make about 9 cups popped popcorn, if prepared in an air popper.

Each serving equals:

DIABETIC: 1 Starch • 1 Fruit • 1 Fat
200 Calories • 4 gm Fat • 3 gm Protein • 38 gm Carbohydrate • 7 mg Sodium • 1 gm Fiber
HE: 1$^1/_3$ Fruit • $^2/_3$ Fat • $^1/_4$ Bread • 17 Optional Calories

Cinnamon Cream Rolls

It's hard to give up those sweet creamy dessert rolls when you decide to live healthier, isn't it? Now you don't have to stop enjoying what you like. These taste so good, friends won't believe how quickly they can be prepared.

✌ Serves 8

1 (8-ounce) can Pillsbury refrigerated crescent dinner rolls
1/2 cup (4 ounces) Philadelphia Fat Free Cream Cheese
1 teaspoon ground cinnamon
2 tablespoons Sugar Twin or Sprinkle Sweet
1/4 cup raisins

Preheat oven to 400 degrees. Spray a cookie sheet with butter-flavored cooking spray. Separate dough into 4 rectangles. In a small bowl, stir cream cheese with a spoon until soft. Spread 2 tablespoons cream cheese over each rectangle. In a small covered container, combine cinnamon and Sugar Twin. Shake well to combine. Evenly sprinkle cinnamon mixture over cream cheese. Sprinkle 1 tablespoon raisins over top of each. Roll each rectangle as for cinnamon rolls. Cut each roll into 4 pieces. Place pieces on prepared cookie sheet. Quickly spray tops of rolls with butter-flavored cooking spray. Bake 7 to 8 minutes or until golden brown. Remove from oven and quickly spray tops again. Place pan on a wire rack and allow to cool completely.

Each serving equals:

DIABETIC: 1 Starch • 1 Fat

134 Calories • 6 gm Fat • 4 gm Protein • 16 gm Carbohydrate • 316 mg Sodium • 1 gm Fiber

HE: 1 Bread • ¼ Protein • ¼ Fruit • 2 Optional Calories

Dilly Corn Muffins

These muffins taste great. The combination of dill and cornmeal is truly delightful.

✌ Serves 8

1 cup all-purpose flour
$^1/_3$ cup yellow cornmeal
2 tablespoons Sugar Twin or Sprinkle Sweet
2 teaspoons baking powder
2 teaspoons dried onion flakes
2 teaspoons dried parsley flakes
1 teaspoon dried dill weed
2 eggs, beaten, or equivalent in egg substitute
2 tablespoons vegetable oil
$^1/_3$ cup skim milk

Preheat oven to 400 degrees. Spray 8 wells of a 12-hole muffin pan with butter-flavored cooking spray or line with paper liners. In a large bowl, combine flour, cornmeal, Sugar Twin, baking powder, onion flakes, parsley flakes, and dill weed. In a small bowl, combine eggs, vegetable oil, and skim milk. Add egg mixture to flour mixture. Mix just to combine. Fill prepared muffin wells $^1/_2$ full. Bake 12 to 15 minutes or until a toothpick inserted in center comes out clean. Place muffin pan on a wire rack and let set 5 minutes. Remove muffins from pan and continue cooling on wire rack.

HINT:

Fill unused muffin wells with water. It protects the muffin tin and ensures even baking.

Each serving equals:

DIABETIC: 1 Starch • 1 Fat

134 Calories • 5 gm Fat • 4 gm Protein • 18 gm Carbohydrate • 95 mg Sodium • 1 gm Fiber

HE: 1 Bread • ¾ Fat • ¼ Protein (limited) • 5 Optional Calories

Lemon Poppy Seed Bread ✳

If you love lemon poppy seed muffins from the bakery but have shied away from them because they are so high in sugars and fats, then try this wonderful bread. By the way, if you want muffins instead of bread, simply spoon the batter into prepared muffin tins instead of the loaf pan.

✌ Serves 12

> 2¼ *cups Bisquick Reduced Fat Baking Mix*
> 1 *(4-serving) package JELL-O sugar-free instant vanilla pudding mix*
> 1 *(4-serving) package JELL-O sugar-free lemon gelatin*
> ⅔ *cup Carnation Nonfat Dry Milk Powder*
> 1 *tablespoon poppy seeds*
> 2 *eggs, slightly beaten, or equivalent in egg substitute*
> 1½ *cups Yoplait plain fat-free yogurt*
> 1 *tablespoon lemon juice*
> ¼ *cup water*
> 1 *teaspoon vanilla extract*

Preheat oven to 350 degrees. Spray a 9-by-5-inch loaf pan with butter-flavored cooking spray. In a large bowl, combine biscuit mix, dry pudding mix, dry gelatin, and dry milk powder. Add poppy seeds. Mix well to combine. In a small bowl, combine eggs, yogurt, lemon juice, water, and vanilla extract. Make a well in center of the dry mixture and add the egg mixture. Mix gently just to combine. Pour batter into prepared pan. Bake 45 to 50 minutes or until a toothpick inserted in center comes out clean. Quickly spray top with butter-flavored cooking spray. Place pan on a wire rack and allow to cool 10 minutes. Remove from pan and continue cooling on rack. Cut into 12 slices.

Each serving equals:

DIABETIC: 1½ Starch

135 Calories • 3 gm Fat • 6 gm Protein • 21 gm Carbohydrate • 420 mg Sodium • 1 gm Fiber

HE: 1 Bread • ⅓ Skim Milk • ¼ Slider • 5 Optional Calories

Zucchini Bread

This is a recipe I made over for a friend. The original was loaded with both sugar and oil. My version is much lighter on both. But Cliff thought it tasted as good or better than any zucchini bread he'd ever tried.

✌ Serves 8 (1 thick or 2 thin slices)

1½ cups all-purpose flour
1 (4-serving) package JELL-O sugar-free instant vanilla pudding mix
¼ cup Sugar Twin or Sprinkle Sweet
1 teaspoon baking soda
1½ teaspoons ground cinnamon
½ teaspoon baking powder
1 cup shredded unpeeled zucchini
½ cup + 1 tablespoon raisins
2 eggs or equivalent in egg substitute
2 tablespoons vegetable oil
1 teaspoon vanilla extract
¾ cup unsweetened applesauce

Preheat oven to 350 degrees. Spray a 9-by-5-inch loaf pan with butter-flavored cooking spray. In a medium bowl, combine flour, dry pudding mix, Sugar Twin, baking soda, cinnamon, and baking powder. Add zucchini and raisins. Mix well to combine. In a small bowl, beat eggs with fork. Add vegetable oil, vanilla extract, and applesauce. Mix well to combine. Stir egg mixture into flour mixture, mixing just until moistened. Pour batter into prepared loaf pan. Bake 50 minutes or until a toothpick inserted in center comes out clean. Cool in pan on a wire rack 5 minutes. Remove from pan and continue cooling on wire rack. Cut into 8 thick or 16 thin slices.

HINT:
   1/4 cup chopped nuts may be stirred in when adding raisins.

Each serving equals:

DIABETIC: 1 Starch • 1 Fat • 1 Fruit

201 Calories • 5 gm Fat • 5 gm Protein • 34 gm Carbohydrate • 434 mg Sodium • 2 gm Fiber

HE: 1 Bread • 3/4 Fat • 3/4 Fruit • 1/4 Protein (limited) • 1/4 Vegetable • 16 Optional Calories

Festive Menus for Family Occasions

If you'd like some help in creating menus using Healthy Exchanges recipes, here are a few suggestions.

A "Welcome to Summer" Family Picnic

A Dinner Party for Friends

A Holiday Buffet by the Fire

Monday Night Football Fest

Index

About the Author

JoAnna Lund, a graduate of the University of Western Illinois, worked as a commercial insurance underwriter for eighteen years before starting her own business, Healthy Exchanges, Inc., which publishes cookbooks, a monthly newsletter, motivational booklets, and inspirational audiotapes. Her first book, *Healthy Exchanges Cookbook*, has more than 250,000 copies in print. Her second book, *HELP: Healthy Exchanges Lifetime Plan*, was published in 1996. A popular speaker with hospitals, support groups for heart patients and diabetics, and service and volunteer organizations, she has appeared on QVC, on hundreds of regional television and radio shows, and has been featured in newspapers and magazines across the country.

The recipient of numerous business awards, JoAnna was an Iowa delegate to the national White House Conference on Small Business. She is a member of the International Association of Culinary Professionals, the Society for Nutrition Education, and other professional publishing and marketing associations. She lives with her husband, Clifford, in DeWitt, Iowa.

I Want to Hear from You. . . .

Besides my family, the love of my life is creating "common folk" healthy recipes and solving every-day cooking questions in *The Healthy Exchanges Way*. Everyone who uses my recipes is considered part of the Healthy Exchanges Family, so please write to me if you have any questions, comments, or suggestions. I will do my best to answer. With your support, I'll continue to stir up even more recipes and cooking tips for the Family in the years to come.

Write to: JoAnna M. Lund
c/o Healthy Exchanges, Inc.
P.O. Box 124
DeWitt, IA 52742

If you prefer, fax me at 319-659-2126 or E-mail me at Healthyjo@aol.com.

The employees of G.K. Hall hope you have enjoyed this Large Print book. All our Large Print titles are designed for easy reading, and all our books are made to last. Other G.K. Hall books are available at your library, through selected bookstores, or directly from us.

For information about titles, please call:

(800) 223-2336

To share your comments, please write:

Publisher
G.K. Hall & Co.
P.O. Box 159
Thorndike, ME 04986